DECISION-MAKING IN
Gastroenterology

EMAD QAYED, MD, MPH

Associate Professor of Medicine
Department of Medicine
Division of Digestive Diseases
Emory University School of Medicine
Chief of Gastroenterology
Grady Memorial Hospital
Atlanta, Georgia

NIKRAD SHAHNAVAZ, MD

Associate Professor of Medicine
Department of Medicine
Division of Digestive Diseases
Emory University School of Medicine
Distinguished Physician
Grady Memorial Hospital
Atlanta, Georgia

ELSEVIER

Elsevier
1600 John F. Kennedy Blvd.
Ste 1800
Philadelphia, PA 19103-2899

DECISION-MAKING IN GASTROENTEROLOGY, FIRST EDITION

ISBN: 978-0-323-93246-2

Executive Content Strategist: Nancy Anastasi Duffy
Content Development Specialist: Kevin Travers
Content Development Manager: Meghan Andress
Publishing Services Manager: Shereen Jameel
Project Manager: Nandhini Thanga Alagu
Design Direction: Renee Duenow

Printed in India

Last digit is the print number: 9 8 7 6 5 4 3 2 1

I dedicate this book to all my trainees, colleagues, and patients, from whom I learn a lot every day. I also dedicate it to my family; my wife Yara and my children Bassem, Zaina, and Mazen.

Emad Qayed

This book would not have been possible without the knowledge I gained from my teachers, colleagues, trainees, and patients. I dedicate this book to all of them as well as to my grandmother Rafat, my parents Roya and Shapour, my wife Suzanne, and our children Andrew and Eliza.

Nikrad Shahnavaz

Contributors

JASNA I. BEARD, MD
Assistant Professor of Medicine
Department of Medicine
Division of Digestive Diseases
Emory University School of Medicine
Atlanta, Georgia

JASON M. BROWN, MD
Associate Professor of Medicine
Senior Physician
Department of Medicine
Division of Digestive Diseases
Emory University School of Medicine
Grady Memorial Hospital Gastroenterology fellowship site director
Atlanta, Georgia

MANJUSHA DAS, MD
Assistant Professor of Medicine
Department of Medicine
Division of Digestive Diseases
Emory University School of Medicine
Atlanta, Georgia

THUY-VAN PHAM HANG, MD
Assistant Professor of Medicine
Department of Medicine
Division of Digestive Diseases
Emory University School of Medicine
Joseph Maxwell Cleland Atlanta VA Medical Center
Decatur, Georgia

ELNAZ JAFARIMEHR, MD
Assistant Professor of Medicine
Senior Physician
Department of Medicine
Division of Digestive Diseases
Emory University School of Medicine
Grady Memorial hospital
Atlanta, Georgia

ANAND JAIN, MD
Assistant Professor of Medicine
Director, Esophageal Disorders Program at the Emory Clinics
Division of Digestive Diseases
Department of Internal Medicine
Emory University School of Medicine
Atlanta, Georgia

VAISHALI PATEL, MD, MHS
Associate Professor of Medicine
Department of Medicine
Division of Digestive Diseases
Emory University School of Medicine
Director of Bariatric Endoscopy, Emory University hospital
Associate Director of Advanced Endoscopy Fellowship Program
Atlanta, Georgia

SRIKRISHNA PATNANA, MD MPH
Assistant Professor
Division of Digestive Diseases
Emory University School of Medicine
Director of Disorders of Gut-Brain Interaction
Grady Memorial Hospital
Atlanta, Georgia

EMAD QAYED, MD, MPH
Associate Professor of Medicine
Department of Medicine
Division of Digestive Diseases
Emory University School of Medicine
Chief of Gastroenterology
Grady Memorial Hospital
Atlanta, Georgia

MOHAMMED A. RAZVI, MD
Assistant Professor of Medicine
Department of Medicine
Division of Digestive Diseases
Emory University School of Medicine
Atlanta, Georgia

GIORGIO ROCCARO, MD, MSCE
Assistant Professor of Medicine
Department of Medicine
Division of Digestive Diseases
Emory University School of Medicine
Atlanta, Georgia

ANAND S. SHAH, MD
Assistant Professor of Medicine
Department of Medicine
Division of Digestive Diseases
Emory University School of Medicine
Director of Hepatology
Joseph Maxwell Cleland Atlanta VA Medical Center
Atlanta, Georgia

NIKRAD SHAHNAVAZ, MD
Associate Professor of Medicine
Department of Medicine
Division of Digestive Diseases
Emory University School of Medicine
Distinguished Physician
Grady Memorial Hospital
Atlanta, Georgia

MICHAEL ANDREW YU, MD, MS
Gastroenterology and Hepatology Fellow
Department of Medicine
Division of Digestive Diseases
Emory University School of Medicine
Atlanta, Georgia

Decision-Making in Gastroenterology

We are excited to present this first edition of "Decision-Making in Gastroenterology". This new book delves into several important topics in gastroenterology and presents them in the form of a flowchart followed by accompanying text. Flowcharts offer many advantages for medical decision-making, whether it is related to the diagnosis of an underlying etiology of a clinical presentation, or to the management of a specific disorder. The visual demonstration of the flowchart can present complex, multi-step information in a clear and organized manner, making it easier to understand the sequence of steps involved in decision-making. Flowcharts also offer a standardized approach to the diagnosis and treatment of gastrointestinal conditions, reducing errors and oversights in decision-making. The accompanying text is divided into paragraphs that correlate with decision points to clarify the specific steps in the medical decision pathway, and to supplement the flowchart with important caveats and considerations.

We acknowledge that the diagnosis and management of many gastrointestinal conditions do not conform to a universal approach that can be summarized in a flowchart. The diagnosis and treatment of gastrointestinal disorders can be complex and should be managed on a case-by-case basis, relying on a physician's experience, patient's preference, and the availability of diagnostic tests and treatment options. In this book, we aim to present an overall framework to provide practical and evidence-based strategies for the diagnosis and treatment of common gastrointestinal disorders. We hope that readers find this book useful in their studies and in clinical practice, and we encourage them to reach out to the authors or to the publisher with any feedback.

EMAD QAYED

NIKRAD SHAHNAVAZ

Acknowledgements

We are fortunate and thankful to work with a diverse group of expert clinicians in the Division of Digestive Diseases at Emory University, who contributed several chapters in this book, and we are grateful for their contribution. We would like to thank Nancy Anastasi Duffy and Kevin Travers for their valuable support in publishing this book.

Contents

PART I
Symptoms and Signs

1 Gastroesophageal Reflux Disease

Jasna I. Beard

Gastroesophageal reflux disease (GERD) is a common complaint in a general gastroenterology clinic and a widespread threat to quality of life in patients of all ages and comorbidities. It consists of the effortless regurgitation or flow of acidic gastric contents into the esophagus or oropharyngeal cavity, often experienced as a burning sensation in the chest, that occurs with sufficient frequency and severity as to impair day-to-day activities.

A. The first and most important step in obtaining a history from a patient reporting reflux symptoms is the exclusion of life-threatening disorders. This risk stratification is most commonly done by assessing for the presence of alarm symptoms, such as unintended weight loss, impaired esophageal transit on swallowing, or evidence of gastrointestinal (GI) blood loss, for example. If any of these signs or symptoms is present, the patient warrants an urgent upper endoscopy. This is often accompanied by additional laboratory and imaging studies.

B. When alarm symptoms are absent but acid reflux is considered, the signs and symptoms can be categorized as typical or atypical. Atypical reflux symptoms include chronic cough, recurrent sinusitis, and chest pressure or pain, for example. If the patient endorses such symptoms, it is important to advise urgent cardiopulmonary evaluation and treat accordingly, if, for example, coronary artery disease is discovered. If the patient's cardiopulmonary evaluation is unrevealing, they may proceed to a trial of proton pump inhibitors (PPIs), alongside those patients with typical GERD symptoms.

C. An 8-week PPI trial is generally advised due to the slow, but lasting, process of decreasing acid production by irreversibly inhibiting the hydrogen-potassium ATPase pump of the gastric parietal cells. If the symptoms substantially improve, an extended course or a temporary increase in dose is considered, alongside lifestyle measures (e.g., decreasing portion sizes, maintaining 3 hours between eating and reclining, quitting tobacco product use, and elevating head of bed). Once the symptoms resolve, a slow weaning process is often recommended in order to avoid rebound acid production. While exact practices can differ widely, it often involves halving the dose of the PPI approximately every 2 weeks, as symptoms permit. The patients may do well with no medications or with a combination of lifestyle modification and as-needed short-acting agents like famotidine or calcium carbonate, for example. On the other hand, if there is no substantial improvement despite the PPI trial, an upper endoscopic exam, with or without confirmatory pH testing, can be considered.

D. An esophagogastroduodenoscopy (EGD) examines the upper GI tract and offers the ability to get biopsies and photo-document the mucosal lining from the esophagus to the third portion of duodenum. In an evaluation of a patient exhibiting symptoms of GERD, it can help exclude typical signs of acid reflux such as moderate to severe reflux esophagitis (Los Angeles grade C or D), Barrett esophagus changes, or peptic esophageal strictures. If these are seen, one can consider continued focus on acid reduction, lifestyle measures, and ancillary medications such as alginates, antihistamines, and neuromodulators. If signs of reflux features are not seen, confirmatory pH testing after discontinuation of acid-reducing medications can be considered and is especially useful in defining the role of acid reflux in patients with atypical symptoms.

E. During pH testing, a wireless pH sensing capsule is attached to the lower esophageal mucosa via suction and provides a report of acid reflux events, while the patient documents symptom events (e.g., heartburn, cough, and chest pain). If the timing of the two events correlates, one can conclude that reflux may be contributing to symptoms and refocus on GERD treatment measures.

F. If the acid reflux and symptom events do not correlate or if acidic gastroesophageal reflux is *not* seen on pH testing, one can consider the possibility of alternative diagnoses. These can include motility disorders (e.g., achalasia, scleroderma, and gastroparesis), bile reflux, functional heartburn, and others. Additional testing and treatment trials are then discussed and can include esophageal and gastric motility studies and use of agents such as tricyclic antidepressants. Of note, a pH study *without* interruption of medical therapy can also be useful in cases of documented and confirmed GERD with incomplete symptom control in order to determine the utility of ongoing acid reflux suppression. If symptom correlation is low, one may focus on treatment of possible overlapping syndromes like functional dyspepsia.

G. Patients with confirmed acid reflux disease whose symptoms remain inadequately controlled with medical management (i.e., lifestyle measures, PPIs, ancillary medications like prokinetics, antihistamines, or alginates) can consider surgical or endoscopic options. These include procedures that augment the gastroesophageal junction pressure, such as endoscopic transoral incisionless fundoplication (TIF), laparoscopically placed magnetic ring system, or surgical partial or circumferential fundoplication. Each option must take into consideration the patient's comorbidities and anatomical factors, such as the presence of hiatal hernia or esophageal dysmotility.

BIBLIOGRAPHY

1. Katz PO, Dunbar KB, Schnoll-Sussman FH, Greer KB, Yadlapati R, Spechler SJ. ACG clinical guideline for the diagnosis and management of gastroesophageal reflux disease. *Am J Gastroenterol.* 2021;117(1): 27-56.
2. Richter JE, Vaezi MF Gastroesophageal reflux disease. Sleisenger and Fordtran's Gastrointestinal and Liver Disease. 11th ed. Elsevier; 2020.

ALGORITHM 1.1 Flowchart for the diagnosis and management of gastroesophageal reflux disease (*GERD*). *EGD,* Esophagogastroduodenoscopy; *ENT,* ear-nose-throat; *GERD,* gastroesophageal reflux disease; *PPI,* proton pump inhibitor.

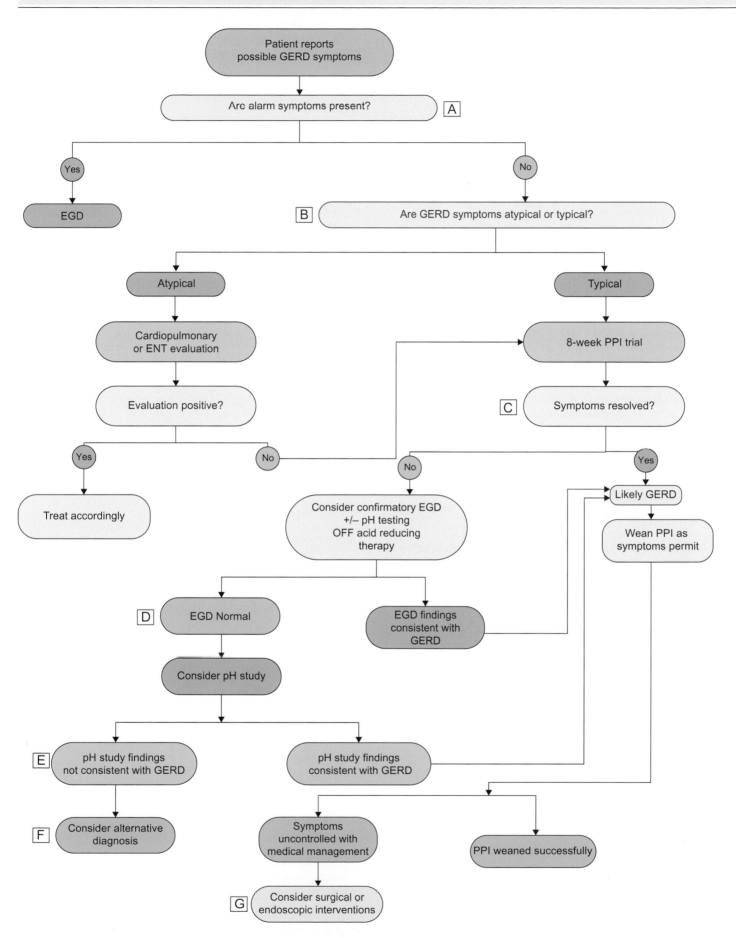

2 Dysphagia

Nikrad Shahnavaz

Dysphagia is the sensation that food is being stalled during its passage from the mouth to the stomach. In evaluating patients with dysphagia, it is essential to obtain a thorough history from the patient. Some patients might initially describe it as pain during swallowing, regurgitation of the food, or even vomiting; however, more meticulous questioning would confirm dysphagia as the principal complaint. The etiology of dysphagia is usually related to mechanical or neurological disorders of the oropharynx or esophagus.

A. Oropharyngeal dysphagia is due to inability to propel the food bolus from the hypopharynx into the esophagus and is usually felt within 1 second after the swallow is initiated. In this condition, the patient is unable to initiate the swallow. It is frequently described as choking or coughing immediately after the attempt to eat.

B. Modified barium swallow or video swallow study is performed by the radiology technician and speech pathologist to evaluate the anatomy and physiology of the oral cavity, hypopharynx, and upper esophageal sphincter during swallow.

C. Common neuromuscular causes of oropharyngeal dysphagia include stroke, Parkinson disease, multiple sclerosis, amyotrophic lateral sclerosis, muscular dystrophy, or thyroid dysfunction. Structural etiologies for oropharyngeal dysphagia are associated with head and neck cancers, radiation, cervical spinal disorders, or Zenker's diverticulum. Oropharyngeal dysphagia should be evaluated by an ear-nose-throat specialist or neurology services based on the etiology.

D. Esophageal dysphagia is described by the patient as hindering of the food bolus at the lower sternum or epigastric region that occurs several seconds after initiation of the swallow.

E. Performing barium swallow before upper endoscopy in all patients is controversial. However, it is proper to selectively perform this test in patients with history of caustic injury, radiation, laryngeal surgery, neck malignancy, or concern for Zenker's diverticulum. These patients may have complex esophageal strictures, and performing the barium swallow provides a map to the esophagus and allows the endoscopist to plan for effective esophageal dilation during endoscopy. Barium swallow can also give a clue to the diagnosis for some esophageal motility disorders such as achalasia (bird's beak appearance) and distal esophageal spasm (corkscrew appearance).

F. Upper endoscopy is the test of choice for esophageal dysphagia. It can diagnose and potentially treat mechanical causes of dysphagia. Esophageal mucosal biopsies are performed to rule out eosinophilic esophagitis.

G. When upper endoscopy is nondiagnostic, if the dysphagia is to both solid and liquid, esophageal motility disorders like achalasia or ineffective esophageal motility are the plausible cause of dysphagia. This diagnosis must be confirmed with esophageal manometry study.

H. In patients with dysphagia to solid foods and normal endoscopy, barium swallow may be useful to exclude small intraluminal abnormalities or extrinsic lesions that could be missed during endoscopy.

I. Patients with dysphagia and unremarkable endoscopy, barium swallow, and esophageal manometry may have gastroesophageal reflux disease (GERD) or esophageal hypersensitivity which usually respond to a trial of acid suppressive therapy.

BIBLIOGRAPHY

1. Liu LWC, Andrews CN, Armstrong D, et al. Clinical Practice Guidelines for the assessment of uninvestigated esophageal dysphagia. *J Can Assoc Gastroenterol.* 2018;1(1):5-19.
2. Malagelada JR, Bazzoli F, Boeckxstaens G, et al. World gastroenterology organization global guidelines: dysphagia—global guidelines and cascades update September 2014. *J Clin Gastroenterol.* 2015;49(5):370-378.
3. Sleisenger and Fordtran's Gastrointestinal and Liver Disease, 11th Edition, Elsevier, 2021. Chapter 13: Symptoms of esophageal disease.

ALGORITHM 2.1 Evaluation of patients with dysphagia. *GERD,* Gastroesophageal reflux disease.

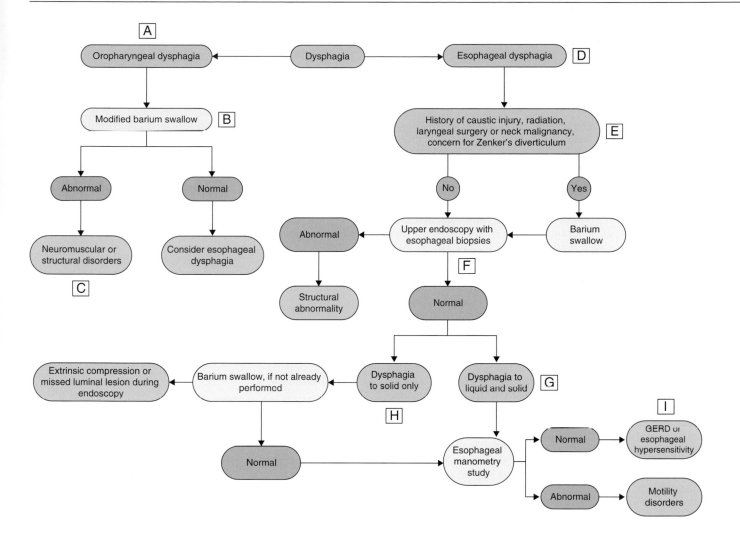

3 Hiccups

Jason M. Brown

Hiccups are the noise produced by a spasm of the diaphragm, causing a quick inhalation that is itself aborted by the rapid closure of the glottis. They are also referred to as "hiccoughs," and the medical term is called "singultus," which is derived from the Latin term "*singult*," that means "to catch one's breath while sobbing." Hiccups can be considered a form of physiologic myoclonus and can occur at a rate of 4–60 hiccups per minute. They are typically caused by diaphragmatic irritation, gastric distension, thoracic or central nervous irritation or tumors, or metabolic derangements such as hypokalemia, hypocalcemia, hyponatremia, and uremia. Spicy foods, smoking, and alcohol can also directly irritate the gastrointestinal (GI) or pulmonary tract; anxiety and stress can also play a role. Hiccups are defined as "persistent" if they last >48 hours, and as "intractable" if they last >1 month.

A. A careful history and physical examination are critical when considering the etiology of hiccups. Asking about gastrointestinal symptoms (dysphagia, heartburn, or abdominal pain), cardiopulmonary symptoms (chest pain or cough), and neurological complaints (headache, dizziness, or focal neurological deficits) may lead to the etiology of the refractory hiccups. Patients should be asked to give a narrative history of the hiccups, including the timing, duration, onset, alleviating factors, and exacerbating factors. Whether the hiccups occur when the patient is sleeping is also important to ascertain. Refractory hiccups due to psychogenic causes (anxiety, malingering, or conversion disorder) usually do not occur while the patient is sleeping. Dietary and social history should be obtained (ask about diet heavy in spicy foods, smoking, and alcohol use). The impact on quality of life is important and should be documented. A careful surgical history can also add to the differential diagnosis if it indicates prior instrumentation in the chest or abdomen. Finally, a careful medication history is vital. Examples of medications that have been associated with hiccups include corticosteroids, benzodiazepines, opioids, barbiturates, antidopaminergics, and chemotherapeutic agents (e.g., carboplatin).

B. If no etiology is clearly suggested by the history and physical examination, a general approach is to check a metabolic panel, obtain a chest x-ray (CXR), and screen for drug and alcohol usage.

C. If a gastrointestinal trigger is suspected, an esophagogastroduodenoscopy (EGD) may be warranted to evaluate for evidence of reflux disease or gastric outlet obstruction. Cross-sectional imaging can be obtained to evaluate for any other structural abnormality of the chest or abdomen that may harbor a trigger.

D. If a central or peripheral neurological etiology is suspected, prompt neurology consultation should be obtained. Head imaging can also be a reasonable next step to evaluate for a mass or other abnormality.

E. If an ear-nose-throat (ENT) etiology is suspected, prompt ENT referral should be made.

F. A trial of twice-daily proton pump inhibitors (PPIs) is a reasonable first pharmacologic step when approaching persistent or intractable hiccups of any etiology.

G. If a PPI trial fails, there are other pharmacologic options to consider:
- First-line therapy: baclofen, gabapentin, or pregabalin
- Second-line therapy: metoclopramide
- Third-line therapy: chlorpromazine
- Other options: amitriptyline, nifedipine, phenytoin, valproate, carbamazepine

H. Nonpharmacologic therapy includes:
- Acupuncture referral
- Hypnosis

I. Surgical therapy incudes referral for consideration of:
- Phrenic nerve ablation
- Cervical epidural block
- Vagal nerve stimulator implantation

BIBLIOGRAPHY

1. Sleisenger and Fordtran's Gastrointestinal and Liver Disease. 11th Edition. 2020. Chapter 13, Symptoms of Esophageal Disease.
2. Quiroga JB, García JU, Guedes JB Hiccups: a common problem with some unusual causes and cures. *Br J Gen Pract*. 2016;66(652):584-586.
3. Cole JA, Plewa MC. Singultus [Updated August 7, 2022]. In: StatPearls [Internet]. Treasure Island (FL): StatPearls Publishing; 2023. Available from: https://www.ncbi.nlm.nih.gov/books/NBK538225/

ALGORITHM 3.1 Flowchart for the workup and management of hiccups. *CT*, Computed tomography; *CXR*, chest x-ray; *EGD*, esophagogastroduodenoscopy; *ENT*, ear-nose-throat; *GI*, gastrointestinal; *PPI*, proton pump inhibitor.

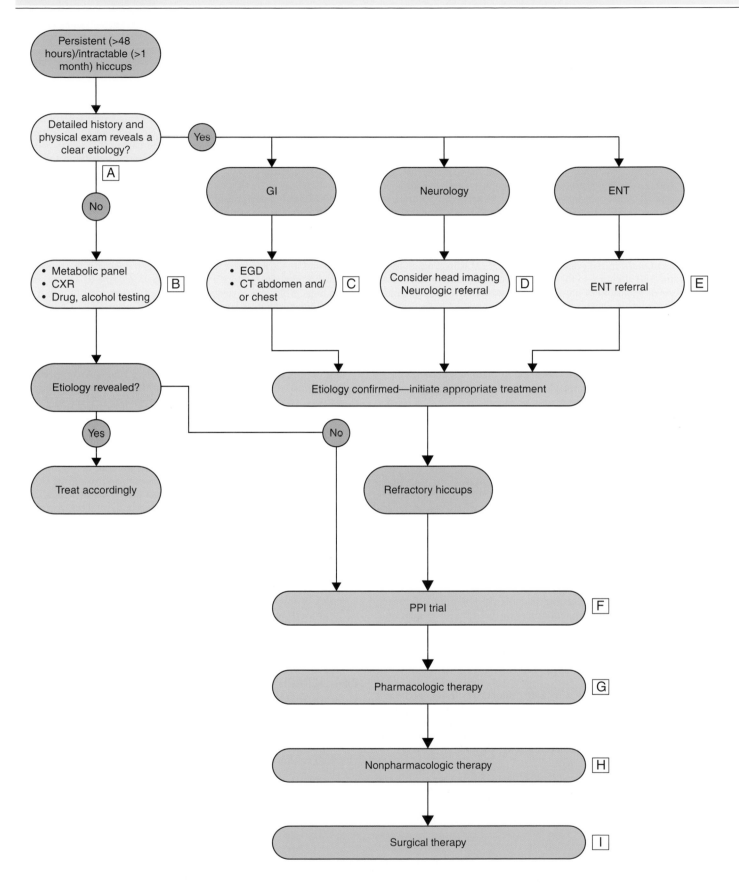

4 Acute Abdominal Pain

Nikrad Shahnavaz

Acute abdominal pain is a frequent complaint that brings patients to emergency room (about 8% of all visits in the United States). Nearly 40% of these visits conclude with nonspecific findings. Of the other 60% in whom a specific etiology is confirmed, most are surgical disorders that warrant further evaluation and intervention. In a smaller portion, life-threatening conditions are present. Therefore, the evaluation of acute abdominal pain must be cost-effective, timely, and accurate so that the treatment of patients who are seriously ill is not hindered and resources are not overutilized on patients with a self-limiting disorder.

A. Identifying the characteristic features of the pain is the most important element of the initial evaluation of the patient with acute abdominal pain. And attention to these features will lead to a rapid clinical diagnosis or exclusion of life-threatening conditions and will guide the subsequent diagnostic testing. These features include location, character, chronicity, intensity, and radiation of the abdominal pain in addition to aggravating and alleviating factors. Physical exam is necessary to detect any evidence of hemodynamic instability, peritonitis, bowel obstruction, acute cholecystitis, acute pancreatitis, or appendicitis. In women with lower abdominal pain, pelvic exam is an essential part of the physical exam.

B. Patients with acute abdominal pain should have laboratory evaluation including complete blood count (CBC), serum chemistries, lactic acid level, urinalysis, liver tests, amylase/lipase, and pregnancy testing (in all women of reproductive age).

C. Lethargy, hypotension, tachycardia, or diaphoresis along with laboratory tests manifesting leukocytosis with left shift, metabolic acidosis, or elevated serum lactate level is associated with tissue hypoperfusion and shock. Patients who present with these findings are likely to require urgent surgical intervention or intensive care.

D. Common characteristics of the history, physical examination, and white blood cell (WBC) count in patients with appendicitis have been used to generate a predictive tool known as the *Alvarado score*. The scoring system includes migration of pain (1 point), anorexia (1 point), nausea (1 point), tenderness in the right lower quadrant (RLQ) (2 points), rebound tenderness (1 point), fever (1 point), leukocytosis (2 points), and left WBC shift (1 point). A score of 4 or lower accurately excludes appendicitis, especially in men. The score is less accurate in women and children.

E. The computed tomography (CT) scan dramatically improves the accuracy of diagnosis in patients with acute appendicitis. An appendix diameter greater than 10 mm, periappendiceal fat inflammation, presence of fluid in the RLQ, and failure of contrast dye to fill the appendix are the diagnostic features of appendicitis in CT scan. To reduce the risk of radiation exposure, some experts recommend RLQ ultrasound (US) instead of CT in children and adolescents. For pregnant patients, magnetic resonance imaging (MRI) has become the imaging method of choice, with comparable sensitivity and specificity to CT scan.

F. Biliary pain is a postprandial pain in the right upper quadrant (RUQ) or epigastric area, caused by transient obstruction of the cystic duct by a gallstone, usually lasting less than 6 hours. Acute cholecystitis is the result of persistent obstruction of the cystic duct by a gallstone so the pain is persistent and could be associated with nausea, vomiting, and low-grade fever. On exam, RUQ tenderness, guarding, and Murphy sign (inspiratory arrest on palpation of the RUQ) are classic findings. Mild leukocytosis and elevated serum total bilirubin and alkaline phosphatase levels are common. During RUQ US, demonstration of gallstones may suggest biliary pain, whereas the finding of stones with gallbladder wall thickening, pericholecystic fluid, and sonographic Murphy sign (pain on compression of the gallbladder with the US probe) is diagnostic of acute cholecystitis. RUQ pain, fever/chills, and jaundice (Charcot triad) are suggestive of ascending cholangitis which needs immediate initiation of intravenous (IV) fluids, antibiotics, and urgent bile duct drainage.

G. In adults, 70% of cases of small bowel obstruction (SBO) are caused by postoperative adhesions. The remainder are usually from incarcerated hernias, inflammatory bowel disease (IBD), or malignancies. The pain in SBO is characterized by sudden onset, cramping, periumbilical abdominal pain, followed by nausea and vomiting. Guarding, localized tenderness, as well as lactic acidosis or leukocytosis could be signs of intestinal ischemia or perforation of the obstructed bowel.

H. Sudden-onset, diffuse or localized sharp abdominal pain, involuntary guarding, and rebound tenderness are usually the signs of peritonitis which can be caused by perforated peptic ulcer disease or diverticulitis. Acute mesenteric ischemia presents with abrupt onset of intense cramping epigastric and periumbilical pain out of proportion to abdominal exam findings. These etiologies must urgently be confirmed with abdominal CT scan with IV contrast with or without oral contrast.

BIBLIOGRAPHY
1. Sleisenger and Fordtran's Gastrointestinal and Liver Disease, 11th Edition, Elsevier, 2020. Chapter 11, Acute abdominal pain.
2. Goldman-Cecil Medicine. Approach to the patient with gastrointestinal disease, 26th Edition, Elsevier, 2019. Chapter 123.

ALGORITHM 4.1 Evaluation of a patient with acute abdominal pain. *AAA,* Abdominal aortic aneurysm; *CT,* computed tomography; *EEG,* electroencephalogram; *EGD,* esophagogastroduodenoscopy; *FAST,* focused abdominal sonogram for trauma; *MRI,* magnetic resonance imaging; *RLQ,* right lower quadrant; *RUQ,* right upper quadrant; *SBO,* small bowel obstruction; *US,* ultrasound.

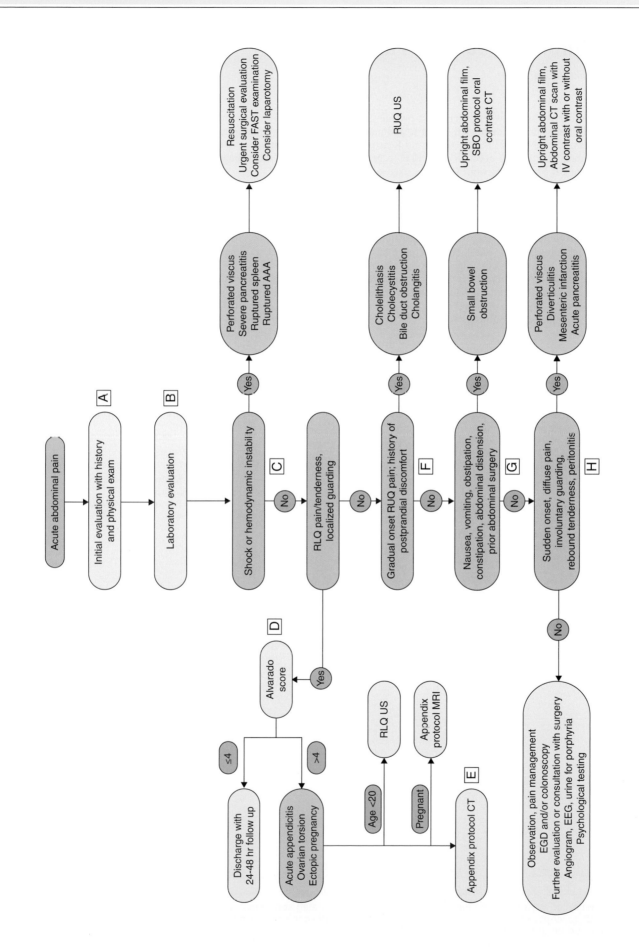

5 Chronic Abdominal Pain

Nikrad Shahnavaz

Abdominal pain is considered chronic when it has been present constantly or intermittently for 6 months or longer. Chronic abdominal pain is a challenging clinical problem for both patients and their physicians. The clinician must differentiate between structural (organic) disorders and disorders of gut-brain interaction (DGBI). A diagnosis of DGBI (formerly known as functional gastrointestinal [GI] disorders) is generally considered once potential causes of organic chronic abdominal pain have been confidently excluded.

A. Like acute abdominal pain, the first step in the evaluation of a patient with chronic abdominal pain is to obtain a detailed history. The characteristic of the pain and any clue suggesting organic disorders are the mainstay of the history in patients with chronic abdominal pain. Presence of alarm features (fever, night sweats, appetite change, weight loss, and nocturnal awakening) suggests organic diseases. Also, physical examination is important to search for evidence of a systemic disease.

B. Chronic abdominal wall pain (CAWP) is the cause of chronic abdominal pain in up to 30% of patients presenting to a gastroenterology clinic with this complaint. Anterior cutaneous nerve entrapment syndrome (ACNES) and myofascial pain syndrome (MFPS) are common causes of CAWP. Recognizing these conditions can avoid further studies or unnecessary surgical intervention. This should be suspected when the abdominal pain is localized and unrelated to eating or bowel movement, but clearly related to movement. During physical examination, tensing the abdominal muscles by the patient causes increased localized tenderness to palpation (*Carnett sign*).

C. Laboratory evaluation must include complete blood count (CBC), serum chemistries, liver tests, amylase/lipase, and urinalysis. If history and physical exam suggest, studies to rule out diabetes, thyroid dysfunction, celiac disease, porphyria, and lead toxicity need to be considered.

D. In young patients with no alarm features or family history of colon cancer or inflammatory bowel disease who show unremarkable routine laboratory evaluation, nonorganic causes of abdominal pain are the most likely diagnosis and further testing should be minimized.

E. In older patients or those with alarming features, it is paramount to confidently exclude organic disorders including malignancy. The workup usually starts with imaging (computed tomography [CT] or magnetic resonance imaging [MRI]) and continues with upper endoscopy, colonoscopy, and other investigations based on their symptoms and findings of the studies.

F. Centrally mediated abdominal pain syndrome (CAPS), formerly known as the functional abdominal pain syndrome, is a distinct medical disorder. This condition relates to central nervous system (CNS) amplification of normal regulatory visceral signals and is characterized by continuous or frequently recurrent abdominal pain that is not related to bowel habits and eating. Patients with CAPS often have a history of anxiety, depression, somatization, posttraumatic stress disorder (PTSD), or sexual and physical abuse. Once the diagnosis of CAPS is made, the primary focus should move away from further testing and toward development of an effective multifaceted treatment plan that incorporates pharmacological and behavioral treatments.

BIBLIOGRAPHY

1. Sleisenger and Fordtran's Gastrointestinal and Liver Disease, 11th Edition, 2020. Chapter 12, Chronic abdominal pain.
2. Goldman-Cecil Medicine, 26th Edition, 2019. Chapter 123, Approach to the patient with gastrointestinal disease.

ALGORITHM 5.1 Evaluation of chronic abdominal pain. *CAPS*, Centrally mediated abdominal pain syndrome; *CT*, computed tomography; *EGD*, esophagogastroduodenoscopy; *EPS*, epigastric pain syndrome; *ERCP*, endoscopic retrograde cholangiopancreatography; *IBS*, irritable bowel syndrome; *RUQ*, right upper quadrant; *SOD*, sphincter of Oddi dysfunction.

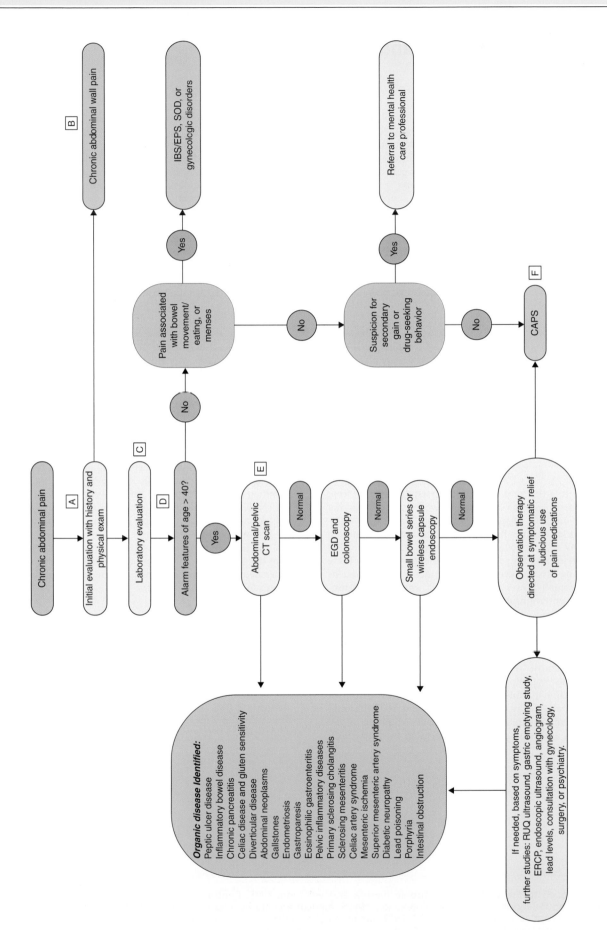

Chronic abdominal pain

A   Initial evaluation with history and physical exam

B   Chronic abdominal wall pain

C   Laboratory evaluation

D   Alarm features or age > 40?

Yes

No

E   Abdominal/pelvic CT scan

Normal

EGD and colonoscopy

Normal

Small bowel series or wireless capsule endoscopy

Normal

Observation therapy directed at symptomatic relief Judicious use of pain medications

Pain associated with bowel movement/ eating, or menses

Yes   IBS/EPS, SOD, or gynecolcgic disorders

No

Suspicion for secondary gain or drug-seeking behavior

Yes   Referral to mental health care professional

No

F   CAPS

Organic disease Identified:
Peptic ulcer disease
Inflammatory bowel disease
Chronic pancreatitis
Celiac disease and gluten sensitivity
Diverticular disease
Abdominal neoplasms
Gallstones
Endometriosis
Gastroparesis
Eosinophilic gastroenteritis
Pelvic inflammatory diseases
Primary sclerosing cholangitis
Sclerosing mesenteritis
Celiac artery syndrome
Mesenteric ischemia
Superior mesenteric artery syndrome
Diabetic neuropathy
Lead poisoning
Porphyria
Intestinal obstruction

If needed, based on symptoms, further studies: RUQ ultrasound, gastric emptying study, ERCP, endoscopic ultrasound, angiogram, lead levels, consultation with gynecology, surgery, or psychiatry.

6 Chronic Nausea and Vomiting

Nikrad Shahnavaz

Nausea is an unpleasant feeling of imminent vomiting. It typically occurs prior to or during vomiting but can happen in isolation. Vomiting refers to the forceful oral expulsion of gastric or intestinal contents that is associated with contraction of the abdominal musculature. Chronic nausea and vomiting is defined by symptom duration of at least 4 weeks. It can result from a variety of gastrointestinal (GI) and non-GI causes.

A. A detailed clinical history and careful physical examination are central to diagnosing the etiology of chronic nausea and vomiting. Symptom characteristics and associated symptoms often suggest a diagnosis. Particular attention should be paid to medication history, especially opiates and cannabinoid use. Signs of weight loss and dehydration should be sought during physical examination. Diagnostic studies for chronic nausea and vomiting should be guided by the history and physical examination.

B. Laboratory tests to order in patients with chronic nausea and vomiting should include a complete blood count, complete metabolic panel, thyroid function tests, hemoglobin A1c, and a pregnancy test in all women of reproductive age. Moreover, serum drug levels and urine drug screening are obtained if there is concern about certain drug toxicity (digoxin, theophylline, or salicylates) or chronic recreational drug use (opiates, cannabis).

C. An important early step in the evaluation of a patient with chronic nausea and vomiting is to identify or exclude GI causes of the symptoms.

D. Forceful expulsion of the food, vomiting of partially digested food an hour after a meal, bilious vomiting, or severe, colicky pain that improves after vomiting suggests mechanical (partial) obstruction as the cause of chronic nausea and vomiting. A succussion splash detected by listening over the epigastrium while shifting the abdomen side to side also suggests gastric outlet obstruction. These patients should be investigated by upper endoscopy followed by upper GI series/small bowel follow-through and cross-sectional imagings with enterography to rule out gastric and intestinal obstruction.

E. When mechanical obstruction or mucosal diseases are excluded, motility disorders such as gastroparesis or achalasia should be considered. The diagnosis of gastroparesis is based on compatible symptoms (early satiety, postprandial abdominal fullness, and bloating), delayed gastric emptying, and the absence of obstruction or mucosal disease. Delayed gastric emptying can be tested by scintigraphy, breath testing, or wireless motility capsule. Vomiting immediately after eating and regurgitation of undigested food may indicate esophageal diseases such as achalasia, Zenker's diverticulum, or esophageal stricture.

F. Chronic nausea and vomiting caused by electrolyte imbalance (uremia, hyponatremia, or hypercalcemia) or endocrine diseases (adrenal insufficiency, ketoacidosis, or hyperthyroidism) usually resolve following the treatment of the underlying condition.

G. Central nervous system (CNS) symptoms such as headache, vertigo, or focal neurologic deficits may indicate a neurologic source for chronic nausea/vomiting and warrant an imaging of the head as well as further evaluation by a neurologist. Migraine, epilepsy, hydrocephalus, pseudotumor cerebri, or brain lesions that compress or irritate the base of the brain may account for chronic nausea and vomiting.

H. When the workup is nondiagnostic, and the history is suggestive, psychiatric diseases (such as anorexia nervosa and bulimia), cyclic vomiting syndrome, and functional vomiting should be considered in the differential diagnosis of chronic vomiting. Cyclic vomiting syndrome is characterized by clustered, recurrent episodes of vomiting (at least three episodes 1 week or more apart in the past year) with absence of vomiting between the episodes. Other milder symptoms can persist between episodes. A personal or family history of migraine is supportive of the diagnosis. Functional vomiting is diagnosed when the symptoms are not cyclical in nature, and other etiologies including eating disorders, rumination, chronic cannabinoid use (cannabinoid hyperemesis syndrome), and organic causes of vomiting have been excluded. Neuromyelitis optica spectrum disorder (NMOSD) is an autoimmune inflammatory CNS syndrome that is associated with serum aquaporin-4 immunoglobulin G antibodies (AQP4-IgG). In addition to optic neuritis and spinal cord disease, it is a rare cause of unexplained chronic nausea, vomiting, and/or hiccups (area postrema syndrome); and these GI symptoms can precede other neurologic manifestations. Diagnosis is with brain MRI and serum AQP4-IgG.

BIBLIOGRAPHY

1. Sleisenger and Fordtran's Gastrointestinal and Liver Disease, 11th Edition, 2020. Chapter 15, Nausea and vomiting.
2. Goldman-Cecil Medicine, 26th Edition, 2019. Chapter 123, Approach to the patient with gastrointestinal disease.
3. Lacy BE, Parkman HP, Camilleri M. Chronic nausea and vomiting: evaluation and treatment. *Am J Gastroenterol.* 2018;113(5):647-659.
4. Wingerchuk DM, Banwell B, Bennett JL, et al. International consensus diagnostic criteria for neuromyelitis optica spectrum disorders. *Neurology.* 2015;85(2):177-189. https://doi.org/10.1212/WNL.0000000000001729.

ALGORITHM 6.1 Approach to the patient with chronic nausea and vomiting. *CNS,* Central nervous system; *CT,* computed tomography; *EGD,* esophagogastroduodenoscopy; *GI,* gastrointestinal; *MALS,* median arcuate ligament syndrome; *MRI,* magnetic resonance imaging; *NMOSD,* neuromyelitis optica spectrum disorder; *NSAID,* nonsteroidal antiinflammatory drug; *PID,* pelvic inflammatory disease; *PUD,* peptic ulcer disease; *SBFT,* small bowel follow-through; *SMA,* superior mesenteric artery; *UGIS,* upper gastrointestinal series.

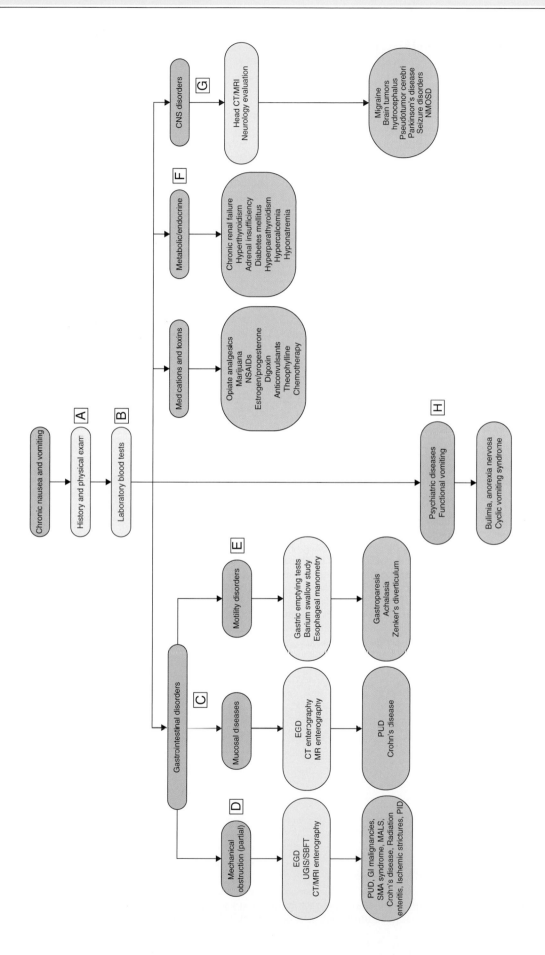

7 Acute Vomiting

Nikrad Shahnavaz

Vomiting is the forceful oral expulsion of gastric contents from retrograde contraction of the duodenum and antrum with compression of the thoracoabdominal musculature. Vomiting may be caused by several gastrointestinal (GI) and non-GI disorders. Most cases of acute vomiting without abdominal pain are self-limited and require no evaluation. On the other hand, acute vomiting with severe abdominal pain could be a sign of serious illness potentially requiring surgical intervention.

A. In all women of reproductive age, pregnancy should be ruled out before any further investigation.

B. Carefully taken history (to identify the potential etiology of vomiting), physical examination (to assess for shock, dehydration, hypotension), and basic laboratory tests including complete blood count (CBC), comprehensive metabolic panel, and serum amylase or lipase levels are the next step of the evaluation for patients with acute vomiting. Severe hyperglycemia may cause acute gastroparesis. Elevated liver or pancreatic enzyme levels suggest hepatobiliary or pancreatic disease.

C. Dehydration, hypotension, and electrolyte abnormalities should be corrected emergently while further investigations are pending to determine the etiology of vomiting.

D. The presence of severe acute abdominal pain along with vomiting usually indicates structural GI disorders such as GI obstruction, hollow viscus perforation, acute pancreatitis, or organ infarction, which need emergent intervention.

E. Peptic ulcer disease, gastric volvulus, paraesophageal hernias, acute and chronic pancreatitis, with associated inflammatory masses or pseudocysts, as well as gastric, duodenal, or pancreatic malignancies are well-described causes of gastric outlet obstruction. Intestinal tumors, adhesions, and intussusception are common causes of acute intestinal obstruction.

F. Perforated viscus or acute appendicitis can cause peritonitis presenting with severe acute abdominal pain and rebound tenderness along with acute nausea and vomiting.

G. Mesenteric ischemia should be considered in elderly patients with vascular disorders and thrombotic diathesis. It may manifest a paucity of physical signs but has a high mortality rate and requires timely management.

H. Patients with acute myocardial infarction (MI) may present with acute-onset vomiting and upper abdominal pain. These atypical symptoms are particularly seen more often in older women and in patients with inferior wall MI.

I. Metabolic and electrolyte disturbances such as hypercalcemia, hyponatremia, hyperglycemia, uremia, and Addison disease can frequently cause nausea and vomiting.

J. Nausea and vomiting are frequent side effects of many common medications such as nonsteroidal antiinflammatory drugs (NSAIDs), antibiotics, cardiovascular drugs (antiarrhythmics), opiates, and azathioprine. Polypharmacy, alcohol use disorder, medication overdose, and acute poisoning can also trigger acute-onset nausea and vomiting.

K. Neurologic and vestibular disorders are common etiologies for acute vomiting (sometimes projectile) and are usually associated with headache, vertigo, or neurological deficits. The list includes vestibular neuritis, labyrinthitis, migraine, meningitis, subdural hematoma, hydrocephalus, intracranial tumors, cerebellar disorders, and temporal lobe epilepsy.

L. Chemotherapy and radiotherapy are well-known causes of nausea and vomiting. Therefore, prophylactic antiemetic therapy is routinely considered. Postoperative (abdominal, gynecologic, eye, and middle ear surgery) vomiting is usually caused by general or epidural anesthesia, ileus, complications of surgery (intestinal perforation, peritonitis), electrolyte abnormalities, or cardiac disease.

BIBLIOGRAPHY

1. Sleisenger and Fordtran's Gastrointestinal and Liver Disease, 11th Edition, 2020. Chapter 15, Nausea and vomiting.
2. Goldman-Cecil Medicine. Approach to the patient with gastrointestinal disease, 26th Edition, Elsevier, 2019. Chapter 123.

ALGORITHM 7.1 Evaluation of patients with acute vomiting. *AXR,* Abdominal x-ray; *CT,* computed tomography; *EGD,* esophagogastroduodenoscopy; *EKG,* electrocardiogram; *ENT,* ear-nose-throat; *GI,* gastrointestinal; *MRI,* magnetic resonance imaging; *RUQ,* right upper quadrant; *US,* ultrasound.

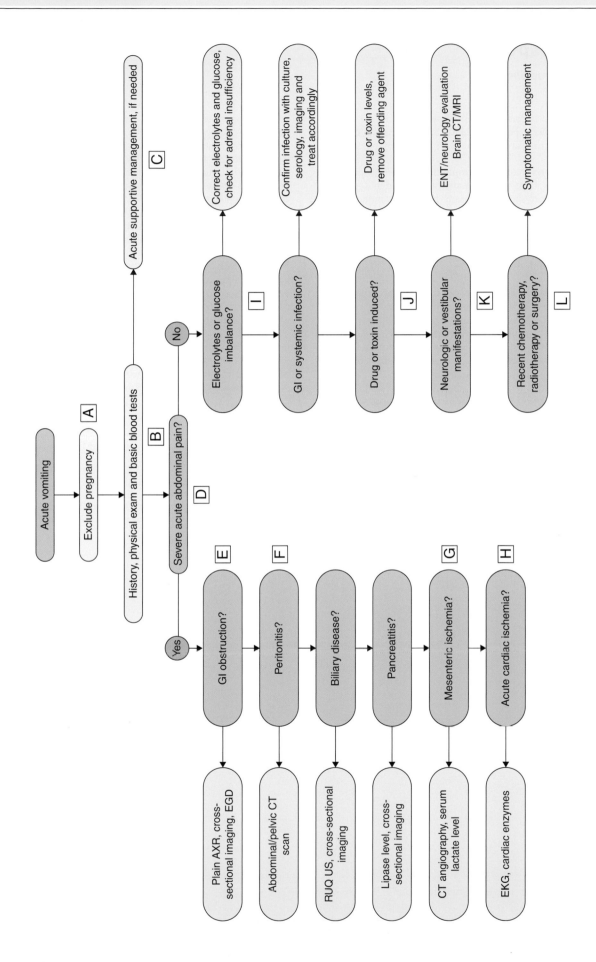

Acute vomiting

Exclude pregnancy A

History, physical exam and basic blood tests B

Severe acute abdominal pain? D

Yes

GI obstruction? E → Plain AXR, cross-sectional imaging, EGD

Peritonitis? F → Abdominal/pelvic CT scan

Biliary disease? → RUQ US, cross-sectional imaging

Pancreatitis? → Lipase level, cross-sectional imaging

Mesenteric ischemia? G → CT angiography, serum lactate level

Acute cardiac ischemia? H → EKG, cardiac enzymes

No

Electrolytes or glucose imbalance? I → Correct electrolytes and glucose, check for adrenal insufficiency

GI or systemic infection? → Confirm infection with culture, serology, imaging and treat accordingly

Drug or toxin induced? J → Drug or toxin levels, remove offending agent

Neurologic or vestibular manifestations? K → ENT/neurology evaluation Brain CT/MRI

Recent chemotherapy, radiotherapy or surgery? L → Symptomatic management

Acute supportive management, if needed C

8 Dyspepsia

Nikrad Shahnavaz

Dyspepsia refers to a heterogeneous group of symptoms in the upper abdomen. Per Rome IV criteria, postprandial fullness, early satiety, epigastric pain, and epigastric burning are four main symptoms of dyspepsia.

A. Uninvestigated dyspepsia refers to symptoms in an individual in whom diagnostic tests have not been performed and no specific diagnosis explaining the dyspeptic symptoms has been identified yet.

B. In patients with dyspepsia who are 60 years old or above, the first step of the management is performing upper endoscopy to rule out gastric malignancy, which is significantly more common in elderly and often can present with dyspepsia.

C. The risk of malignancy in a person with dyspepsia who is younger than 60 years old is very low. Therefore, routine endoscopy is not indicated. However, in a selected group of patients with alarming features such as >5% weight loss, gastrointestinal (GI) bleeding, unexplained anemia, dysphagia, persistent vomiting, lymphadenopathy, or significant family history of GI cancer, endoscopy must be considered early during workup of dyspepsia.

D. Patients with dyspepsia and normal endoscopy and those who are symptomatic despite being negative for *Helicobacter pylori* are diagnosed as functional dyspepsia. According to Rome IV criteria, functional dyspepsia is further classified into two subgroups of postprandial distress syndrome (meal-related dyspepsia) and epigastric pain syndrome (meal unrelated).

E. After discontinuing nonsteroidal antiinflammatory drugs (NSAIDs) and dietary modification, the first line of pharmacologic treatment for patients with functional dyspepsia is a trial of proton pump inhibitors (PPIs) once daily for 4–8 weeks.

F. In refractory cases of epigastric pain syndrome after 4–8 weeks, PPI needs to be stopped and tricyclic antidepressants (TCAs) like low-dose amitriptyline can be tried for 8–12 weeks. The functional dyspepsia treatment trial showed that amitriptyline (50 mg at night) is efficacious in functional dyspepsia compared to the two other treatment arms (escitalopram 10 mg and placebo). Adequate response was seen in 40% of placebo, 53% of amitriptyline, and 38% of escitalopram ($PP = 0.05$). Patients with epigastric pain were more likely to respond to amitriptyline compared to those with dysmotility-type symptoms (early satiety, bloating, and nausea).

G. In patients with postprandial distress syndrome, a trial of prokinetics like metoclopramide for 4 weeks is a reasonable next step after failure of response to PPIs. Other acceptable drug options for refractory postprandial distress syndrome include mirtazapine and buspirone, which can alleviate weight loss and early satiety, respectively.

H. Routine study of gastric motility is not recommended in patients with functional dyspepsia. However, gastric emptying study should be ordered in selected cases with nausea/vomiting predominant symptoms and in patients with known risk factors for gastroparesis.

BIBLIOGRAPHY

1. Sleisenger and Fordtran's Gastrointestinal and Liver Disease. 11th Edition, 2020. Chapter 14, Dyspepsia.
2. Moayyedi P, Lacy BE, Andrews CN, Enns RA, Howden CW, Vakil N. ACG and CAG clinical guideline: management of dyspepsia. *Am J Gastroenterol.* 2017;112(7):988-1013.
3. Talley NJ, Locke GR, Saito YA, et al. Effect of amitriptyline and escitalopram on functional dyspepsia: a multicenter, randomized controlled study. *Gastroenterology.* 2015;149(2):340-49.e2.

ALGORITHM 8.1 Evaluation and management of dyspepsia. *PPI,* Proton pump inhibitor; *TCA,* tricyclic antidepressant.

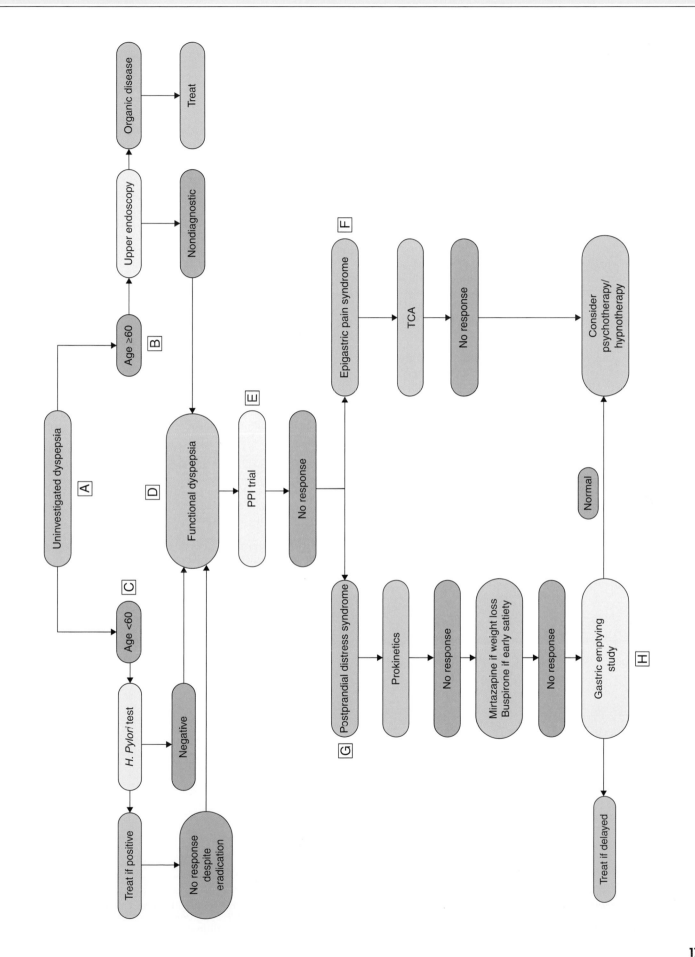

9 Jaundice

Emad Qayed

Jaundice refers to the yellow discoloration of the skin, sclerae, and mucous membranes. This occurs due to elevated plasma bilirubin level resulting in tissue deposition of bilirubin. Bilirubin is produced by heme degradation and circulates the plasma by noncovalently binding to albumin. This unconjugated bilirubin undergoes uptake into the hepatocyte, conversion to conjugated bilirubin (bilirubin monoglucuronide and diglucuronide), and active excretion into the biliary canaliculi and the bile duct. Increased bilirubin production (e.g., hemolysis) or decreased excretion (e.g., biliary obstruction) results in hyperbilirubinemia and jaundice.

A. The initial evaluation of a patient with jaundice should begin with a careful history and physical examination, and basic laboratory studies including complete blood cell count, hepatic panel (total and conjugated plasma bilirubin concentration, aminotransferase levels, alkaline phosphatase levels), and international normalized ratio (INR).

B. Hypercarotenemia is an uncommon condition that causes yellow discoloration of the skin, most prominently in the palms and plantar sides of feet, but not the sclerae. It is caused by excessive consumption of fruits and vegetables containing high levels of carotene such as broccoli, sweet potatoes, carrots, oranges, cantaloupe, red and yellow peppers, apricots, and squash. The serum bilirubin level is normal, while serum beta-carotene levels are elevated. The condition resolves with the decrease in consumption of carotene.

C. Unconjugated hyperbilirubinemia is caused by increased bilirubin production (hemolysis, ineffective erythropoiesis, resorption of hematomas) or decreased conjugation (Gilbert and Crigler-Najjar syndromes, physiologic jaundice of the newborn, and use of protease inhibitors such as indinavir and atazanavir). Gilbert syndrome is a relatively common cause of mild unconjugated hyperbilirubinemia that can worsen with fasting and acute illness.

D. Liver imaging is needed in cases of conjugated hyperbilirubinemia. Liver ultrasound is an excellent test to diagnose cholelithiasis, but it is less sensitive for choledocholithiasis. Nevertheless, it can demonstrate liver lesions, and biliary ductal dilation suggestive of biliary obstruction.

E. If biliary obstruction is suspected, further imaging with computed tomography (CT) or magnetic resonance imaging (MRI)/magnetic resonance cholangiopancreatography (MRCP) is considered if the etiology is unclear. Alternatively, management can proceed with endoscopic retrograde cholangiopancreatography (ERCP) for therapeutic decompression. Endoscopic ultrasound (EUS) is also considered to obtain tissue sampling of peripancreatic or perihepatic masses. Percutaneous transhepatic cholangiography (PTC) can be performed if ERCP is not successful or in cases of severe suprahilar obstruction.

F. If a liver mass is diagnosed without biliary obstruction, then transcutaneous liver mass biopsy is performed to obtain a tissue diagnosis.

G. If cirrhosis is diagnosed, then further workup should focus on finding the etiology of cirrhosis (alcoholic, viral, nonalcoholic steatohepatitis, autoimmune, etc.), consideration of treatment (e.g., antivirals, steroids), and management of complications (ascites, encephalopathy, variceal bleeding).

H. If liver morphology is normal, and there is no biliary obstruction, other etiologies of jaundice and elevated liver enzymes should be considered, such as acute hepatitis A and B, chronic hepatitis B and C, sepsis-induced cholestasis, drug-induced liver injury, autoimmune hepatitis, and primary biliary cholangitis.

I. If the etiology of jaundice remains unclear, with persistent hyperbilirubinemia, then a liver biopsy is required for further diagnosis of underlying liver disease.

ALGORITHM 9.1 Flowchart for the workup and diagnosis of a patient with jaundice. *CBC*, Complete blood count; *CT*, computed tomography; *ERCP*, endoscopic retrograde cholangiopancreatography; *EUS*, endoscopic ultrasound; *MRCP*, magnetic resonance cholangiopancreatography; *MRI*, magnetic resonance imaging; *PTC*, percutaneous transhepatic cholangiography; *US*, ultrasound.

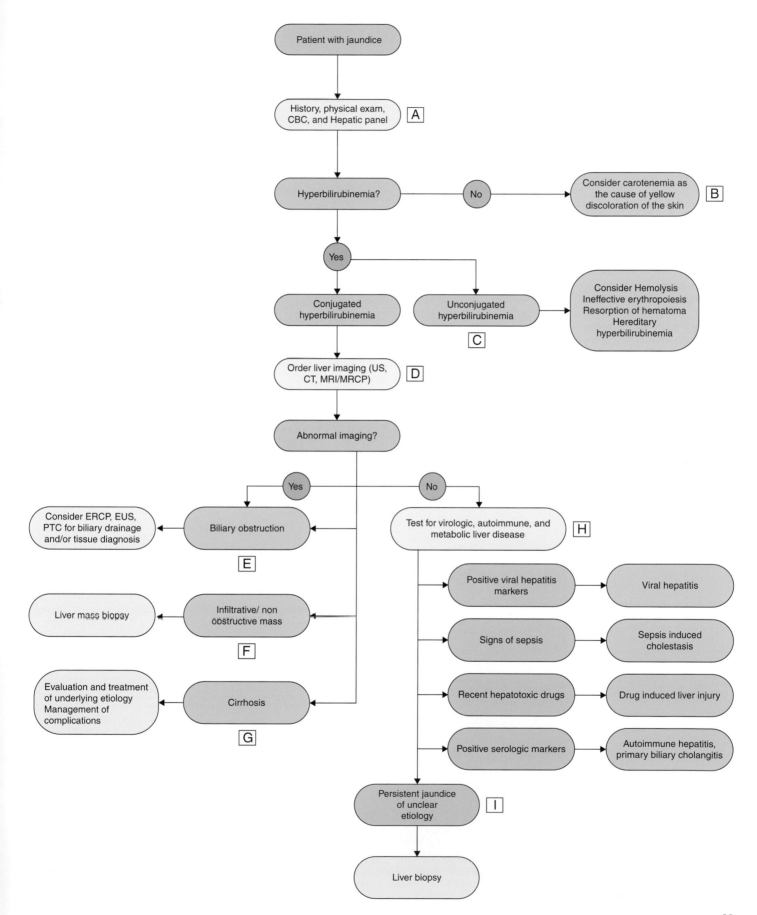

10 Abnormal Weight Loss

Nikrad Shahnavaz

The involuntary loss of more than 5% of baseline weight within 6 to 12 months is clinically important and frequently due to a serious underlying medical or psychiatric illness. Weight loss is often revealed during the clinical evaluation of other medical complaints. Common causes of weight loss in the elderly are depression, dementia, difficulty with chewing or swallowing, malignancy, medications, alcoholism, or limitations in ability to prepare meals. In young patients, weight loss is more frequently due to eating disorders, endocrine disorders, or chronic gastrointestinal (GI) conditions such as inflammatory bowel disease (IBD) or celiac disease. In about a quarter of patients, no cause of weight loss is found.

A. The cause of weight loss is usually suggested from the history and physical examination. Special attention needs to be made to any evidence of anxiety, depression or dementia, drug use, dehydration, or malnutrition, as well as any GI complaint. Alarm features like dysphagia, vomiting, altered bowel habits, jaundice, GI bleeding, or hemoptysis, when present, will direct the next step of the evaluation.

B. Volitional causes, including change of diet or dieting, medications, drug use disorder, increased exercise, eating disorders, or social limitations, should be identified and resolved. Weight status should be reassessed in 1–3 months.

C. Initial laboratory tests include complete blood count (CBC), electrolytes, creatinine, glucose, ferritin, liver enzymes, albumin, calcium, C-reactive protein (CRP), thyroid function tests, and HIV serology. In patients older than 40 years, smokers, or patients with any respiratory symptom, chest x-ray should also be part of the initial workup.

D. Unintentional weight loss associated with anorexia and varying degrees of cachexia is seen with advanced malignancy, chronic infections (HIV or tuberculosis), heart failure, chronic kidney disease, cirrhosis, chronic obstructive pulmonary disease (COPD), adrenal insufficiency, substance use disorder, dementia, or depression. The workup should be directed to identify these etiologies.

E. Weight loss despite normal or increased appetite occurs in the setting of either increased metabolism and energy expenditure (endocrine disorders, such as poorly controlled diabetes, hyperthyroidism, or pheochromocytoma) or GI disorders that disrupt the food digestion/absorption within the small intestines (like IBD, celiac disease, chronic pancreatitis, protein-losing enteropathy, or severe small intestinal bacterial overgrowth).

F. GI diseases that cause mechanical obstruction or dysmotility in the esophagus (cancer, achalasia), stomach (cancer, peptic ulcer disease with gastric outlet obstruction, gastroparesis), small intestine (Crohn's disease, small intestinal dysmotility), or arterial circulation (chronic mesenteric ischemia) may cause weight loss as a result of dysphagia, vomiting, or postprandial pain that limits the ability of the patient to ingest sufficient calories despite having normal appetite.

BIBLIOGRAPHY

1. Sleisenger and Fordtran's Gastrointestinal and Liver Disease, 11th Edition, 2020.
2. Goldman-Cecil Medicine. Approach to the patient with gastrointestinal disease, 26th Edition, Elsevier, 2019. Chapter 123.

ALGORITHM 10.1 Evaluation of a patient with abnormal weight loss. *COPD*, Chronic obstructive pulmonary disease; *CT*, computed tomography; *CXR*, chest radiograph; *EGD*, esophagogastroduodenoscopy; *EMS*, esophageal motility study; *EUS*, endoscopic ultrasound; *GES*, gastric emptying study; *HIV*, human immunodeficiency virus; *PFT*, pulmonary function test; *PTH*, parathyroid hormone; *TFTs*, thyroid function tests; *tTG*, tissue transglutaminase.

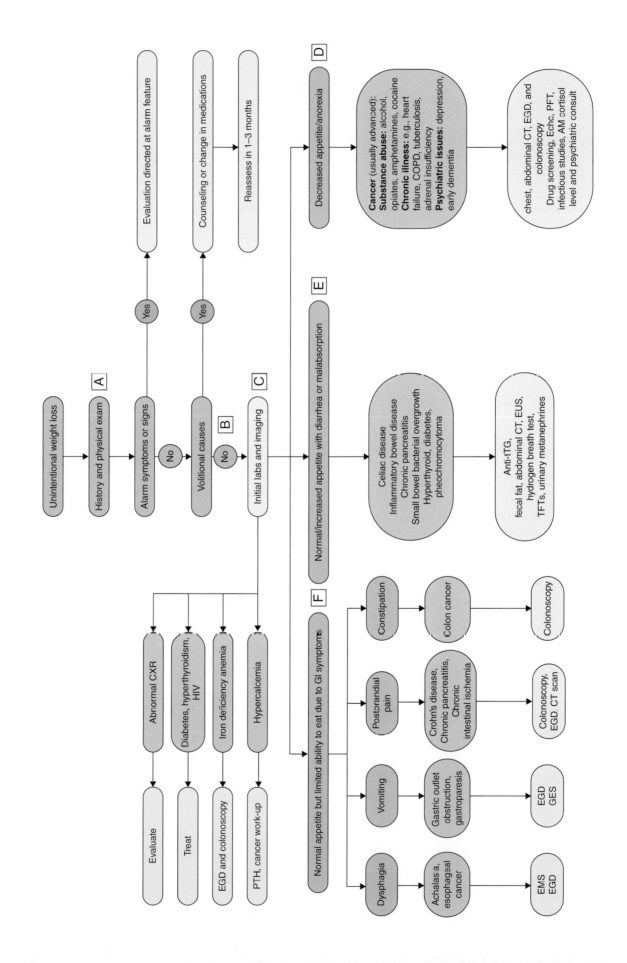

11 Acute Diarrhea

Nikrad Shahnavaz

Acute diarrhea is defined as an abrupt onset of three or more loose or liquid stools above baseline rate, in a 24-hour period, lasting less than 14 days. Persistent diarrhea is typically defined as diarrhea lasting between 14 and 30 days and should be worked up by microbiological assessments, then treated with antimicrobial agents based on the study results.

A. Most individuals with acute diarrhea can keep up with fluids and salt by consumption of water, sports drinks, juice, soup, and saltine crackers. In the adult population, this regimen is recommended over oral rehydration solutions (ORSs). Patients with severe dehydration, suggested by orthostatic hypotension, dry mucous membranes, reduced skin turgor, or altered mental status as well as patients who cannot tolerate oral hydration may need to be admitted and started on intravenous (IV) fluids.

B. Detailed history and physical examination are essential for individuals with acute diarrhea. It includes frequency and characteristics of bowel movements, blood in the stool, duration of the diarrhea, other symptoms like fever, abdominal pain, nausea, vomiting, and any evidence of severe dehydration (reduced or dark urine, dry mucosa, confusion, or dizziness). Travel history, food exposure, new medications especially antibiotics, and any comorbidity including immunosuppression are an important part of history that would guide the management plan.

C. Traditional methods of diagnosis (bacterial culture, microscopy with and without special stains and immunofluorescence, and antigen testing) do not reveal the etiology of most cases of acute diarrheal infection. If available, multiplex polymerase chain reaction (PCR) methods that are Food and Drug Administration (FDA) approved and culture independent should be utilized for the diagnosis of infectious etiologies of diarrhea. These tests can detect a multitude of gastrointestinal pathogens (bacteria, viruses, parasites) in patients with acute and chronic diarrhea. Performance of these tests is of particular importance in immunosuppressed patients who may have opportunistic infections and have higher risk of complications and mortality from any infection (e.g., patients with human immunodeficiency virus with CD4 count less than 200 cells/mm^3, active inflammatory bowel disease, and history of organ transplantation or hematologic malignancy).

D. The severity of acute diarrhea is categorized as mild (no change in activities); moderate (able to function but with forced change in activities due to illness); and severe (total disability due to diarrhea).

E. The evidence does not support empiric use of antibiotic therapy for acute diarrhea, except in case of moderate to severe travel diarrhea when the likelihood of bacterial infection is high. Epidemiological studies demonstrated that most community-acquired diarrhea is viral in etiology (norovirus, rotavirus, and adenovirus). A single dose of azithromycin 1000 mg or 500 mg daily for 3 days is the treatment of choice for travel diarrhea. However, fluoroquinolones (single dose or 3-day course) and rifaximin for 3 days are both effective antibiotic regimens in shortening the duration of illness in travel diarrhea.

F. In patients with non-travel-associated diarrhea who have high-grade fever or dysenteric diarrhea, it is recommended to complete the microbiological assessment first and then start antimicrobial therapy directed by the test results. This approach is particularly important in reducing the risk of complications from Shiga-like toxin–producing *Escherichia coli* (hemolytic uremic syndrome), nontyphoidal Salmonella strains (prolonged intestinal carriage), and *Clostridioides difficile*–associated colitis development.

BIBLIOGRAPHY

1. Riddle MS, DuPont HL, Connor BA. ACG clinical guideline: diagnosis, treatment, and prevention of acute diarrheal infections in adults. *Am J Gastroenterol.* 2016;111(5):602-622. https://doi.org/10.1038/ajg.2016.126.
2. Sleisenger and Fordtran's Gastrointestinal and Liver Disease, 11th Edition, Elsevier, 2021. Chapter 16, Diarrhea.

ALGORITHM 11.1 Management of acute diarrhea. *O&P*, Ova and parasites; *PCR*, polymerase chain reaction

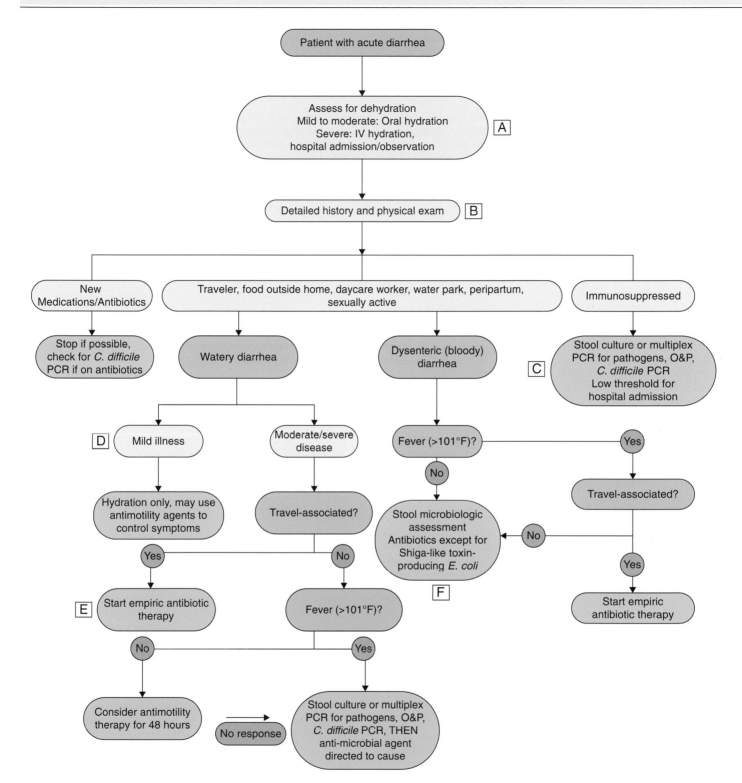

12 Chronic Diarrhea

Nikrad Shahnavaz

Diarrhea could be described as some or all the following changes of bowel habit in an individual: (1) three or more bowel movements a day, (2) more frequent bowel movements than normal for the individual, (3) loose/watery stool, (4) more than 200 g of stool during 24 hours in Western countries, or (5) Bristol stool scale of 6 or 7. Chronic diarrhea refers to persistent symptoms that last more than 4 weeks. Chronic diarrhea is most commonly caused by noninfectious etiologies.

A. The first step in the evaluation of a patient with chronic diarrhea is obtaining a detailed history and physical exam, which can frequently identify the most common etiologies. Special attention needs to be paid to associated symptoms (fecal incontinence, abdominal pain, and alarming features like weight loss and rectal bleeding), coexisting systemic diseases (diabetes, thyroid disease), surgical history (cholecystectomy, intestinal resection), diet, and medications.

B. Fecal incontinence, especially in the elderly population, can masquerade as chronic diarrhea. This needs to be ruled out with a careful history and performing a digital rectal exam. Iatrogenic diarrhea from drugs, surgery, or radiation can be ruled out with reviewing the patient's chart. Irritable bowel syndrome (IBS) and functional diarrhea can be diagnosed based on Rome IV criteria, and in the absence of any alarming feature, no further workup is indicated. Small intestinal bacterial overgrowth (SIBO), food intolerance, and bile malabsorption are three common causes of chronic diarrhea, which can be empirically treated when suspected and in the absence of any alarming feature. Age-appropriate screening colonoscopy must be done in all patients at the age of 45 years old or above.

C. The basic lab tests to be considered in a patient with chronic diarrhea include complete blood count (CBC), comprehensive metabolic panel (CMP), celiac panel, C-reactive protein (CRP), fecal occult blood test, fecal leukocyte or fecal lactoferrin/calprotectin, qualitative stool fat, in addition to bacterial culture, *Clostridioides difficile* testing, and ova/parasite exam, giardia, and cryptosporidium antigens or polymerase chain reaction (PCR) assays.

D. At this juncture, patients with persistent and refractory diarrhea without a clear diagnosis will need colonoscopy to examine the mucosa of the colon and terminal ileum. Random colon biopsies should be obtained to examine for microscopic colitis. In addition, computed tomography (CT) or magnetic resonance imaging (MRI) scan of the abdomen/pelvis with enterography should be considered to rule out structural diseases such as inflammatory bowel disease, gastrointestinal (GI) malignancy, pancreatic disease, bowel ischemia, and diseases of small bowel like obstruction, diverticulosis, or fistula. Upper endoscopy with small bowel biopsies often is done at this stage, although its diagnostic yield is debated in the absence of markers of celiac disease.

E. If structural diseases are ruled out, quantitative analysis of the stool can be used to guide further classification of the chronic diarrhea. That includes measurement of stool sodium and potassium concentration to calculate fecal osmotic gap, stool pH, osmolality, and 24-hour (or 72-hour) stool fat collection. If there is concern about surreptitious laxative use, stool can be analyzed for the concentration of polyethylene glycol, sulfate, phosphate, and magnesium. *Fecal osmotic gap* is calculated as $290 - 2 (Na + K)$. A large gap ($>100\,mOsm/kg$) suggests osmotic diarrhea, and a small gap ($<50\,mOsm/kg$) is suggestive of secretory diarrhea. Negative osmotic gap indicates ingestion of poorly absorbed anions (phosphate or sulfate laxatives). Actual measurement of stool osmolality is used to detect contamination by water or urine ($<290\,mOsm/kg$).

F. Osmotic diarrhea with elevated fecal osmotic gap has a limited differential diagnosis which consists of either ingestion of osmotic laxatives or carbohydrate malabsorption. A fecal pH lower than 6 points toward carbohydrate malabsorption, which can be further confirmed with careful review of the diet and/or lactose hydrogen breath test.

G. Steatorrhea is defined as detection of more than 7 g of fat in the stool over 24 hours after a 3-day diet of 100-g fat daily prior to the collection. However, fat excretion between 7 and $14\,g/24$ hours has a low specificity for fat malabsorption.

H. Secretory diarrhea with small fecal osmotic gap has a long list of differential diagnosis, which includes IBS, functional diarrhea, microscopic colitis, antibiotics use, SIBO (less severe cases), stimulant laxative use, idiopathic secretory diarrhea, adrenal insufficiency, hyperthyroidism, diabetes, chronic intestinal infections, bile acid malabsorption (BAM), and quite rare endocrine tumors such as gastrinoma, VIPoma, or carcinoid tumor. Failure to make a diagnosis by this point is more likely due to overlooking a common cause rather than missing a rare cause of chronic diarrhea. Therefore, it is imperative to review the previous studies and medication list again at this stage.

I. Diarrhea caused by an endocrine tumor is extremely rare. The pretest probability of having these tumors in a patient with chronic diarrhea is so low that ordering endocrine tumor panels in every patient with chronic secretory diarrhea would result in many false-positive results and unnecessary studies. Therefore, testing should only be done in patients with chronic diarrhea and clinical manifestations of a tumor syndrome such as flushing, headache, urticaria pigmentosa, right-sided heart murmur, wheezing, or multiple GI ulcerations.

J. Opiate antidiarrheals such as loperamide are the mainstay of symptomatic management of persistent chronic diarrhea when specific treatment is not possible. Dosing should be scheduled rather than as needed. Empiric trials of bile acid binders (cholestyramine), water-soluble fibers (psyllium), and food exclusion diet (low FODMAP diet) are reasonable approaches in the appropriate clinical settings.

BIBLIOGRAPHY

1. Schiller LR, Pardi DS, Sellin JH. Chronic diarrhea: diagnosis and management. *Clin Gastroenterol Hepatol.* 2017;15:182-192.
2. Schiller LR. Evaluation of chronic diarrhea and irritable bowel syndrome with diarrhea in adults in the era of precision medicine. *Am J Gastroenterol.* 2018;113(5):660-669.
3. Sleisenger and Fordtran's Gastrointestinal and Liver Disease, 11th Edition, Elsevier, 2021. Chapter 16, Diarrhea.

ALGORITHM 12.1 Evaluation and management of patients with chronic diarrhea. *5HIAA,* 5-Hydroxyindoleacetic acid; *CT,* computed tomography; *EGD,* esophagogastroduodenoscopy; *IBS,* irritable bowel syndrome; *MRI,* magnetic resonance imaging; *PEG,* polyethylene glycol; *SIBO,* small intestinal bacterial overgrowth; *VIP,* vasoactive intestinal peptide.

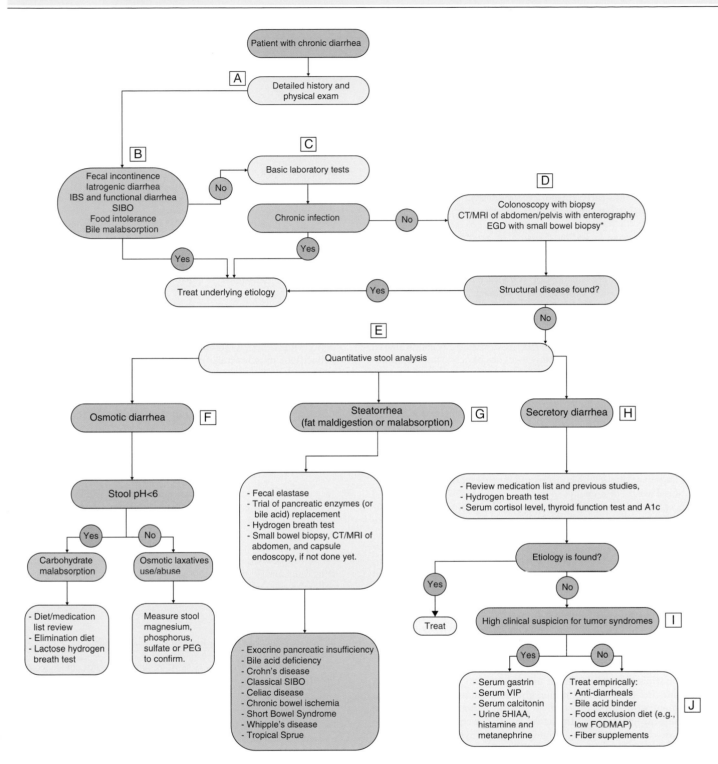

Patient with chronic diarrhea

A — Detailed history and physical exam

B — Fecal incontinence
Iatrogenic diarrhea
IBS and functional diarrhea
SIBO
Food intolerance
Bile malabsorption

No → C — Basic laboratory tests

Chronic infection

Yes

D — Colonoscopy with biopsy
CT/MRI of abdomen/pelvis with enterography
EGD with small bowel biopsy*

No

Structural disease found?

Yes → Treat underlying etiology

Yes

No

E — Quantitative stool analysis

F — Osmotic diarrhea

G — Steatorrhea
(fat maldigestion or malabsorption)

H — Secretory diarrhea

Stool pH<6

Yes → Carbohydrate malabsorption
- Diet/medication list review
- Elimination diet
- Lactose hydrogen breath test

No → Osmotic laxatives use/abuse
Measure stool magnesium, phosphorus, sulfate or PEG to confirm.

- Fecal elastase
- Trial of pancreatic enzymes (or bile acid) replacement
- Hydrogen breath test
- Small bowel biopsy, CT/MRI of abdomen, and capsule endoscopy, if not done yet.

- Exocrine pancreatic insufficiency
- Bile acid deficiency
- Crohn's disease
- Classical SIBO
- Celiac disease
- Chronic bowel ischemia
- Short Bowel Syndrome
- Whipple's disease
- Tropical Sprue

- Review medication list and previous studies,
- Hydrogen breath test
- Serum cortisol level, thyroid function test and A1c

Etiology is found?

Yes → Treat

No → I — High clinical suspicion for tumor syndromes

Yes → - Serum gastrin
- Serum VIP
- Serum calcitonin
- Urine 5HIAA, histamine and metanephrine

No → Treat empirically:
- Anti-diarrheals
- Bile acid binder
- Food exclusion diet (e.g., low FODMAP)
- Fiber supplements — J

13 Constipation

Nikrad Shahnavaz

The American College of Gastroenterology (ACG) defines constipation as "unsatisfactory defecation" characterized by either infrequent stools (fewer than three bowel movements per week) or difficult stool passage (straining, incomplete evacuation, hard/lumpy stools, prolonged defecation, or need for manual maneuvers). Chronic constipation is diagnosed when symptoms of constipation are experienced for at least 3 months, and it is divided into three categories: slow-transit constipation, normal-transit constipation, and defecatory disorder.

A. A detailed history including duration of symptoms, frequency of bowel movements, associated symptoms, and warning features is essential. New-onset constipation may indicate a structural disease, while a long-standing constipation refractory to conservative treatments is suggestive of a functional colorectal disorder. Past medical history including obstetric, surgical, and neurological histories is especially important. Perianal and rectal examination is the most important part of evaluating a patient with constipation, and one should look for anal fissure, external hemorrhoids, rectal prolapse, fecal impaction, rectal mass, or any evidence of pelvic floor dysfunction.

B. Medications that can frequently cause chronic constipation include opioids, calcium or iron supplement, calcium channel blockers, antacids, diuretics, nonsteroidal antiinflammatory drugs (NSAIDs), anticonvulsants, and anticholinergic agents such as antiparkinsonian drugs, antipsychotics, antispasmodics, and tricyclic antidepressants.

C. Red flags in a patient with constipation include rectal bleeding, unintentional weight loss, change in the caliber of stool, severe abdominal pain, or family history of colon cancer. A colonoscopy is recommended only when these alarming features exist or as an age-appropriate screening colonoscopy in all patients above the age of 45 years old. Additional tests include complete blood count (CBC), inflammatory markers (erythrocyte sedimentation rate [ESR] or C-reactive protein [CRP]), biochemical tests (such as thyroid function, serum calcium or glucose levels), and cross-sectional imaging.

D. Initial treatment of constipation should be based on nonpharmacologic interventions including increased physical activity and fluid intake as well as increased fiber intake through dietary modifications or use of soluble fiber supplements (such as psyllium).

E. The pharmacological treatment for constipation usually starts with osmotic laxatives (polyethylene glycol or lactulose). Short-term treatment with stimulant laxatives such as bisacodyl is appropriate as a second-line therapy. The newer agents for constipation include chloride channel activator (lubiprostone), guanylate cyclase C agonists (linaclotide or plecanatide), 5-HT 4 agonist (prucalopride), and sodium-hydrogen exchanger 3 inhibitor (tenapanor). These drugs may be considered in different dosages when lifestyle modifications and osmotic and stimulant laxatives do not provide adequate relief of constipation.

F. In patients with refractory constipation despite trying different classes of laxatives, physiologic studies including anorectal manometry, balloon expulsion test, and defecography are indicated to assess for defecatory disorder. Per Rome criteria, to diagnose dyssynergic defecation, a combination of two of the following three abnormal tests of the pelvic floor is required on attempted defecation: (1) impaired evacuation on balloon expulsion or defecography; (2) inappropriate contraction of the pelvic floor muscles on manometry or defecography; and (3) inadequate propulsive forces as assessed by manometry or defecography.

G. The defecation retraining including optimal posture for defecation (raising the feet above floor level when using a Western-type toilet), along with anorectal biofeedback (to train the patients to relax their pelvic floor muscles during straining and to coordinate this relaxation with abdominal maneuvers to boost entry of stool into the rectum), has been proved effective in the treatment of constipation due to defecatory disorder. A trial of glycerin or bisacodyl suppositories, or enemas (by liquifying the impacted stool) may be effective in dyssynergic defecation. Surgical repair of rectocele or prolapse is considered in patients who have evidence of retained contrast during defecography or women who require digital vaginal pressure to relieve the constipation.

H. In patients with normal defecation physiology and refractory constipation, assessment of colonic transit time is important to confirm slow-transit constipation. Three recommended methods to evaluate the colonic transit time include radiopaque markers, wireless motility capsule, and colonic transit scintigraphy. In selected cases with refractory slow-transit constipation, surgical options with subtotal colectomy and ileorectal anastomosis are considered after excluding generalized intestinal dysmotility or pseudo-obstruction syndrome.

BIBLIOGRAPHY

1. Sleisenger and Fordtran's Gastrointestinal and Liver Disease, 11th Edition, Elsevier, 2021. Chapter 19: Constipation.
2. Chang L, Sultan S, Lembo A, et al. AGA clinical practice guideline on the pharmacological management of irritable bowel syndrome with constipation. *Gastroenterology*. 2022;163(1):118-136.
3. American Gastroenterological Association Bharucha AE, Dorn SD, Lembo A, Pressman A. American Gastroenterological Association medical position statement on constipation. *Gastroenterology*. 2013;144(1):211-217.
4. Paquette IM, Varma M, Ternent C, et al. The American Society of Colon and Rectal Surgeons' clinical practice guideline for the evaluation and management of constipation. *Dis Colon Rectum*. 2016;59(6):479-492.

ALGORITHM 13.1 Evaluation and management of chronic constipation. *MR*, Magnetic resonance.

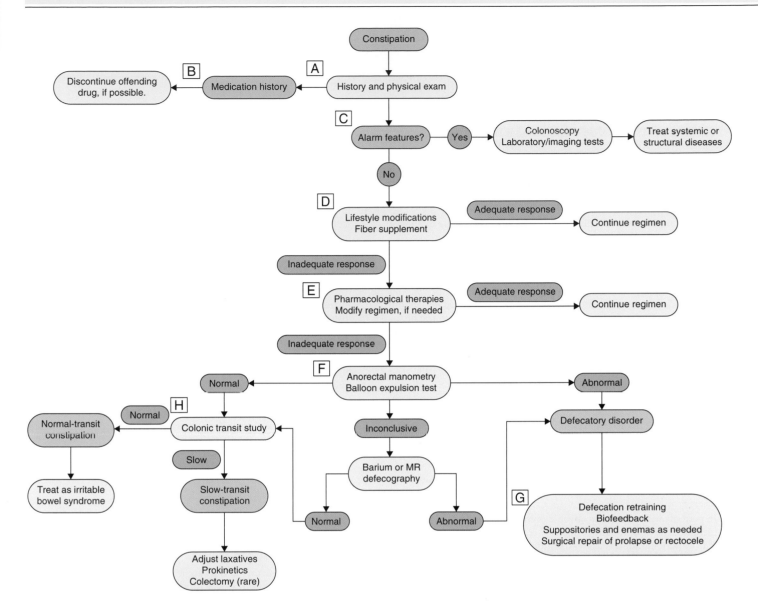

14 | Fecal Incontinence

Emad Qayed

Fecal incontinence is a common clinical problem in which the patient is unable to control the passage of feces or gas through the anus, leading to involuntary leakage of fecal content. Normal continence requires a structurally and functionally intact anorectal unit (rectum, internal and external anal sphincter, and puborectalis muscle). Any disease that causes structural or neural damage to these structures can result in fecal incontinence.

A. Fecal incontinence can cause significant reduction in the quality of life and may lead to patient embarrassment and reluctance to discuss the clinical problem with healthcare providers. Patients may describe fecal incontinence as loose stools or diarrhea. Therefore, it is important to obtain a careful history and ask specific questions about the ability to control bowel movements. The history should ask about coexisting chronic diarrhea, constipation, fecal impaction, rectal bleeding, surgical history (hemorrhoidectomy, obstetric history including the use of forceps delivery and episiotomy), history of diabetes, urinary incontinence, spinal cord trauma, pelvic radiation, and drugs that can alter stool characteristics and muscle tone (anticholinergics, antidepressants, laxatives, muscle relaxants). Physical examination should focus on the anorectal area by careful inspection for hemorrhoids, skin tags and excoriations, and rectal prolapse. Perianal sensation should be examined by gently stroking the perianal skin. This maneuver should lead to contraction of the external anal sphincter, indicating a normal anocutaneous reflex (anal wink). Absence of this reflex suggests neuronal injury. The digital rectal exam is performed using a lubricated gloved index finger to assess the internal anal sphincter by evaluating the resting anal tone, and the external anal sphincter by evaluating the "squeeze" pressure.

B. In patients with coexisting chronic diarrhea, further evaluation may include stool studies and endoscopy (refer to Chapter 12). In those with functional diarrhea, treatment with loperamide and other antidiarrheals may lead to significant improvement in diarrhea and incontinence.

C. Patients with severe constipation may experience anal fissures, leading to impaired anal sensation and passive incontinence. In addition, prolonged retention of stool due to incomplete evacuation may lead to impaired rectal sensation, and prolonged relaxation of the internal anal sphincter, leading to fecal seepage.

D. Anorectal disorders are important risk factors for fecal incontinence. Hemorrhoids, anal fissures, perianal fistulae, rectal prolapse, and proctitis can impair perianal sensation and sphincter function.

E. Careful identification of coexisting diarrhea, constipation, and anorectal disorders, combined with appropriate medical and/or surgical treatment, is key to resolving fecal incontinence. In patients who improve, clinical follow-up is suggested as appropriate. If fecal incontinence persists despite appropriate therapy, then further anorectal motility testing is appropriate.

F. In patients without significant coexisting diarrhea, constipation, or anorectal disorders, further testing with anorectal manometry is recommended.

G. Anorectal manometry is useful to provide clues to the underlying etiology of incontinence. It provides important information about the functional integrity of the internal and external anal sphincters. In addition, it measures rectal sensation and the ability to feel rectal distension and the urge to defecate.

H. Patients with decreased rectal sensation or those with normal manometry may benefit from several interventions such as stool bulking agents (antidiarrheals, fiber supplements), pelvic floor biofeedback, sphincter augmentation with injectable bulking agents, or sacral nerve stimulation.

I. Patients with weak internal or external anal sphincter may benefit from endoanal ultrasound to further characterize the anal sphincters. This test evaluates sphincter integrity and thickness, and detects sphincter defects and/or presence of muscle atrophy. Magnetic resonance imaging (MRI) is an alternative imaging test to examine the anal sphincters.

J. Patients with documented anal sphincter defects may benefit from anal sphincter repair, sphincter augmentation with injectable bulking agents, or sacral nerve stimulation.

K. Patients with refractory and severe fecal incontinence should be considered for an ileostomy or colostomy.

BIBLIOGRAPHY

1. Wald A, Bharucha AE, Limketkai B, et al. ACG clinical guidelines: management of benign anorectal disorders. *Am J Gastroenterol.* 2021;116(10):1987–2008.

ALGORITHM 14.1 Flowchart for the workup and management of a patient with fecal incontinence. *MRI,* Magnetic resonance imaging.

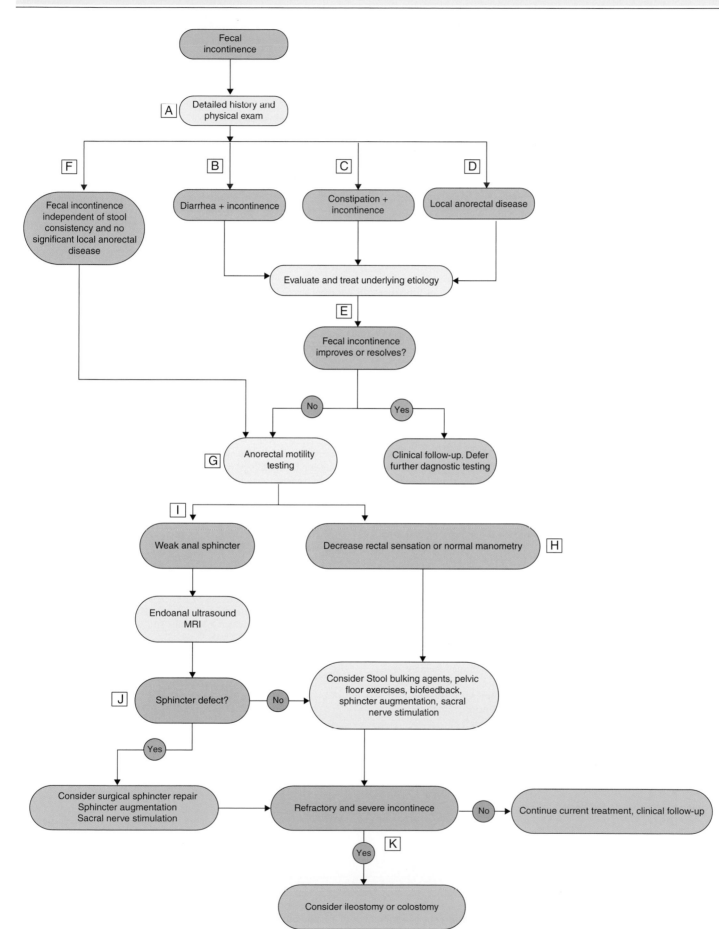

15 Upper Gastrointestinal Bleeding

Emad Qayed

Upper gastrointestinal bleeding (UGIB) refers to bleeding from the upper gastrointestinal tract, from a location accessible by the standard gastroscope (up to the second portion of the duodenum). Significant UGIB presents with hematemesis, melena, or hematochezia.

A. Patients with suspected UGIB should undergo a complete history and physical examination. Important elements in the history include the type and volume of bleeding, gastrointestinal signs and symptoms (dysphagia, abdominal pain, vomiting), significant previous medical history (peptic ulcer disease, liver and cardiopulmonary disease), medication history, and alcohol use. Physical exam should focus on assessing vital signs, mental status, and presence of active bleeding from a nasogastric tube or from the rectum. Abdominal exam should elicit any signs of surgical abdomen, for which further immediate surgical consultation is warranted.

B. Laboratory tests, including type and cross-match, complete blood count, and chemistry panels, should be performed in all patients with significant UGIB.

C. Ongoing resuscitation includes intravenous (IV) fluids and transfusion of packed red blood cells to maintain a hemoglobin level of 7 g/dL. A threshold of 8 g/dL is recommended for patients with preexisting cardiovascular heart disease.

D. Patients with suspected or known cirrhosis should receive IV octreotide and antibiotics. IV proton pump inhibitor (PPI) is given prior to endoscopy, which decreases the likelihood of encountering active bleeding or a visible vessel during esophagogastroduodenoscopy (EGD) and may allow for earlier hospital discharge. In patients with severe bleeding, consider IV erythromycin, IV metoclopramide, or nasogastric tube to decrease the amount of blood in the stomach and improve visualization during EGD.

E. Patients with large-volume hematemesis and/or altered mental status should undergo endotracheal intubation to protect the airway and prevent aspiration.

F. EGD should be performed within 24 hours of hospital presentation in most patients with nonvariceal UGIB. If variceal UGIB is suspected, then EGD should be performed within 12 hours of presentation. Endoscopic findings will dictate the next steps in management.

G. Patients with peptic ulcer disease and either active bleeding or a visible nonbleeding vessel should undergo endoscopic therapy, followed by high-dose IV PPI for 48–72 hours to decrease the risk of rebleeding. If an ulcer with overlying clot is identified, then aggressive irrigation or suction to expose and treat the underlying lesion should be performed. If the clot cannot be removed, consider epinephrine injection in high-risk patients. These patients should also receive IV PPI and close monitoring after the EGD. Patients with peptic ulcer disease with a clean ulcer bed or pigmented spot do not need endoscopic therapy and can be given oral PPI and discharged within 24 hours if they are stable otherwise.

H. During EGD, the endoscopist should consider performing a gastric ulcer biopsy to rule out malignancy, and a gastric biopsy to rule out *Helicobacter pylori*. If this is not done, other tests for *H. pylori* should be performed, and a repeat EGD in 6–8 weeks should be considered to document ulcer healing.

I. Patients with esophageal variceal bleeding are treated with endoscopic variceal band ligation. Octreotide is continued for 3–5 days depending on the severity of the underlying liver disease, and antibiotics are continued for 7 days. EGD should be repeated every 2–8 weeks to ablate the esophageal varices, followed by periodic EGD for variceal surveillance.

J. Other common etiologies of UGIB that are treated endoscopically are Mallory Weiss tears and arteriovenous malformation. Gastric varices can be treated with endoscopic injection with cyanoacrylate glue, or by radiologic procedures such as balloon occluded retrograde transvenous obliteration (BRTO) or transjugular intrahepatic portosystemic shunt (TIPS).

K. If EGD does not reveal a source of bleeding in a patient with confirmed melena or hematochezia, then workup should proceed to rule out colonic or small bowel bleeding.

BIBLIOGRAPHY

1. Laine L, Barkun AN, Saltzman JR, Martel M, Leontiadis GI. ACG Clinical Guideline: Upper Gastrointestinal and Ulcer Bleeding. [published correction appears in Am J Gastroenterol. 2021 Nov 1;116(11):2309]. *Am J Gastroenterol.* 2021;116(5):899–917.
2. Henry Z, Patel K, Patton H, Saad W. AGA Clinical Practice Update on Management of Bleeding Gastric Varices: Expert Review. *Clin Gastroenterol Hepatol.* 2021;19(6):1098–1107.e1. https://doi.org/10.1016/j.cgh.2021.01.027.

ALGORITHM 15.1 Flowchart for the workup and management of a patient with suspected upper gastrointestinal bleeding. *CBC,* Complete blood count; *EGD,* esophagogastroduodenoscopy; *IV,* intravenous; *NPO,* nil per os; *PPI,* proton pump inhibitors.

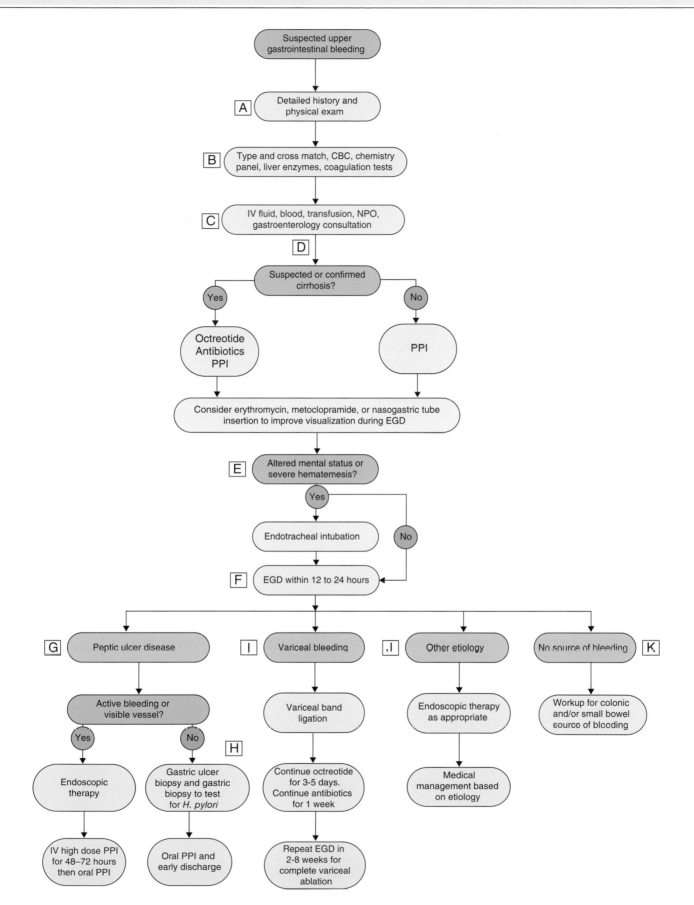

16 Severe Hematochezia

Emad Qayed

Hematochezia refers to the passage of bright red blood per rectum, and it usually results from a colonic source of bleeding. However, severe upper gastrointestinal or small bowel bleeding can also lead to severe hematochezia. The management of mild hematochezia without hemodynamic instability consists of basic history and physical examination (including anorectal exam), blood count, and referral for elective outpatient colonoscopy. Severe hematochezia with ongoing bleeding requires hospital admission, resuscitation, and more urgent management. Most cases of severe hematochezia are caused by diverticular disease and angiectasia. Less common etiologies include ischemic colitis, Dieulafoy's lesion, radiation proctopathy, or iatrogenic bleeding (post polypectomy, postsurgical anastomotic bleeding).

A. Patients with severe hematochezia should undergo a complete history and physical examination. Important elements in the history include the volume of bleeding, presence of gastrointestinal symptoms (abdominal pain, weight loss), significant comorbidities (cardiovascular disease, peptic ulcer disease, liver disease), and medication history. A recent colonoscopy with polypectomy raises the suspicion of postpolypectomy bleeding. Physical exam should focus on assessing vital signs, mental status, and presence of active bleeding. An abdominal examination should look for signs of tenderness, which may indicate the presence of colitis, and rectal exam should examine for any obvious anorectal sources of bleeding. Laboratory tests, including type and cross-match, blood count, and chemistry panels, should be performed on all patients with severe hematochezia. Resuscitation measures include intravenous fluids and transfusion of packed red blood cells to maintain a hemoglobin level of 7–9 g/dL. Patients with known cardiovascular disease should receive a blood transfusion if the hemoglobin falls below 8 g/dL, to maintain a hemoglobin level of 8–10 g/dL.

B. Patients who are hemodynamically unstable after initial resuscitation should undergo computed tomography angiography (CTA) to further evaluate the site of bleeding.

C. If a source of bleeding is identified on CTA, further management usually includes angiography and transarterial embolization. If a bleeding source within reach of the endoscopy is found (e.g., duodenal or rectal), then endoscopy is performed if the patient has become hemodynamically stable.

D. If a source of bleeding is not identified on CTA, and the patient has become hemodynamically stable, then esophagogastroduodenoscopy (EGD) and colonoscopy should be performed for further evaluation. If a source of bleeding is identified, endoscopic therapy should be performed. If a source of bleeding is not identified, then workup for suspected small bowel bleeding should be pursued.

E. If a source of bleeding is not identified on CTA, and the patient remains hemodynamically unstable due to continued bleeding, then conventional angiography or emergency laparotomy should be considered for further management of refractory profuse bleeding.

F. Patients who are hemodynamically stable after initial resuscitation should receive colonic preparation and undergo colonoscopy during their hospital stay. It is not clear if early colonoscopy (within 24 hours) improves important outcomes compared to later colonoscopy. Unprepped colonoscopy or flexible sigmoidoscopy should be avoided. If a source of bleeding is identified, endoscopic therapy should be performed. In patients with concurrent known cirrhosis or history of peptic ulcer disease, an EGD can be performed before or concurrently with the initial colonoscopy (not shown in the algorithm).

G. If a source of bleeding is not identified on colonoscopy, EGD or push enteroscopy should be performed to rule out an upper gastrointestinal source of bleeding. If a source of bleeding is identified, endoscopic therapy should be performed. If a source of bleeding is not identified, then workup for suspected small bowel bleeding should be pursued (see Chapter 17).

BIBLIOGRAPHY

1. Qayed E, Dagar G, Nanchal RS. Lower gastrointestinal hemorrhage. *Crit Care Clin.* 2016;32(2):241–254. https://doi.org/10.1016/j.ccc.2015.12.004.PMID: 27016165.
2. Triantafyllou K, Gkolfakis P, Gralnek IM, et al. Diagnosis and management of acute lower gastrointestinal bleeding: European Society of Gastrointestinal Endoscopy (ESGE) Guideline. *Endoscopy.* 2021;53(8):850–868. https://doi.org/10.1055/a-1496-8969. Erratum in: Endoscopy. 2021 Jun 17; PMID: 34062566.
3. Sengupta N, Feuerstein JD, Jairath V, et al. Management of patients with acute lower gastrointestinal bleeding: an updated ACG guideline. *Am J Gastroenterol.* 2023;118(2):208–231. https://doi.org/10.14309/ajg.0000000000002130.

ALGORITHM 16.1 Flowchart for the workup and management of a patient with severe hematochezia. *CBC,* Complete blood count; *CT,* computed tomography; *EGD,* esophagogastroduodenoscopy; *IV,* intravenous fluids; *NPO,* nil per os.

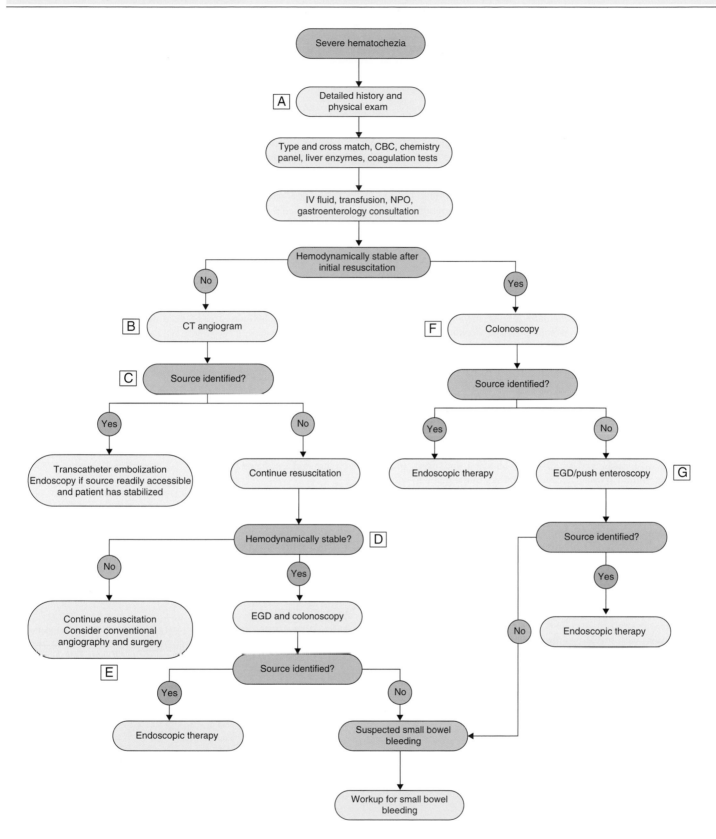

17 Suspected Small Bowel Bleeding

Emad Qayed

Small intestinal bleeding is suspected in patients with overt bleeding (melena, hematochezia) or occult bleeding (iron deficiency anemia) with unrevealing upper and lower endoscopic examination. There are several endoscopic and radiologic tests to investigate the source of small intestinal bleeding. These include video capsule endoscopy (VCE), push enteroscopy, deep enteroscopy (single balloon, double balloon, or spiral enteroscopy), computed tomographic enterography (CTE), magnetic resonance enterography, computed tomographic angiography (CTA), tagged red blood cell (RBC) scintigraphy, Meckel's scan, and surgery with intraoperative enteroscopy.

A. In patients with suspected small intestinal bleeding, a second-look upper and/or lower endoscopy should be considered if the previous endoscopies were incomplete and an upper or lower gastrointestinal (GI) source of bleeding is suspected. Commonly missed lesions include peptic ulcer disease, Dieulafoy lesions, and angiectasia. If a second-look endoscopy is unrevealing, further workup for small bowel bleeding depends on the severity of bleeding.

B. In patients with suspected occult small intestinal bleeding (e.g., iron deficiency anemia), it is reasonable to treat with iron replacement therapy and monitor response to treatment. In patients who do not respond to iron replacement therapy, VCE should be performed. Some physicians would proceed directly to VCE for further workup (see Chapter 18—Iron Deficiency Anemia).

C. Patients with suspected small bowel bleeding and overt, profuse bleeding should receive hemodynamic resuscitation with intravenous fluids and transfusion of packed RBCs.

D. If the patient remains unstable, then workup should proceed with conventional angiography, and transarterial embolization should be performed if a source is identified.

E. If a source is not identified, and the patient remains unstable, then further management with surgery and intraoperative enteroscopy should be considered. If the patient becomes stable, then further workup with VCE and deep enteroscopy should be considered.

F. If a patient with initial profuse bleeding becomes stable after initial resuscitation efforts, further workup with tagged RBC scintigraphy or CTA is reasonable. If a source is identified, conventional angiography and transcatheter embolization should be performed. If a source is not identified, then further workup should proceed with VCE.

G. Patients with suspected small bowel bleeding and overt subacute ongoing bleeding should undergo VCE for further workup. If a small bowel source of bleeding is identified on VCE, deep enteroscopy should be performed to reach the site of bleeding and apply therapeutic interventions to achieve hemostasis, or to perform a biopsy of the lesion. The location of the small bowel bleeding will dictate the approach of deep enteroscopy. Anterograde enteroscopy should be performed if the lesion is within the proximal 60% of the small intestine, while retrograde enteroscopy is performed if the lesion is within the distal 40% of the small bowel. Patients with suspected small bowel obstruction should not undergo VCE.

H. If the VCE does not reveal a source of bleeding, then the condition can be classified as "obscure overt GI bleeding." These patients have a source of bleeding that could not be identified anywhere in the GI tract, and the actual source of bleeding could be within or outside of the small bowel.

I. In patients with obscure overt bleeding and suspicion of upper or lower source of bleeding, repeat upper or lower endoscopy should be performed.

J. If there is ongoing suspicion of small bowel bleeding, small bowel imaging with (CTE or magnetic resonance enterography [MRE]) should be performed. In young patients with obscure overt bleeding, a Meckel's scan should be performed to rule out Meckel's diverticulum and associated bleeding.

K. On rare occasions in which the source of bleeding remains obscure despite multiple tests, pharmacologic provocation (with heparin and clopidogrel) followed by angiography can be considered. Intraoperative enteroscopy an invasive surgery in which a laparotomy and enterotomy are performed, followed by the passage of an endoscope through the enterotomy to examine the small bowel. This should be reserved for patients with continued obscure overt GI bleeding.

BIBLIOGRAPHY

1. Gerson LB, Fidler JL, Cave DR, Leighton JA. ACG clinical guideline: diagnosis and management of small bowel bleeding. *Am J Gastroenterol.* 2015;110(9):1265–1287. quiz 1288. doi: 10.1038/ajg.2015.246. PMID: 26303132.

ALGORITHM 17.1 Flowchart for the workup and management of a patient with suspected small intestinal bleeding. *CTA,* Computed tomographic angiography; *CTE,* computed tomographic enterography; *EGD,* esophagogastroduodenoscopy; *MRE,* magnetic resonance enterography; *RBC,* red blood cell; *VCE,* video capsule endoscopy.

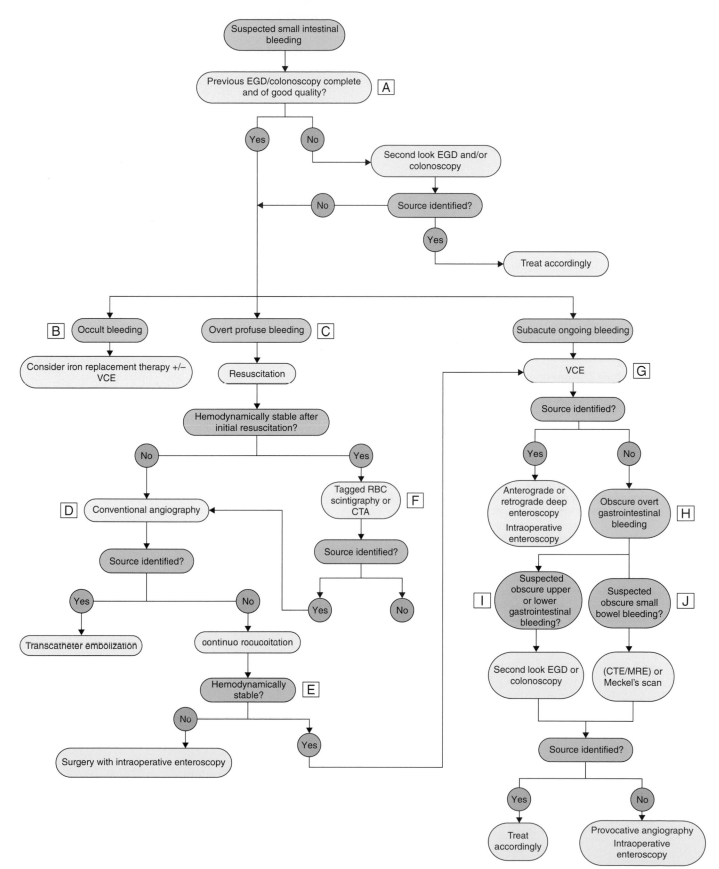

18 Iron Deficiency Anemia

Emad Qayed

Iron deficiency anemia may result from decreased oral intake of iron (e.g., malnutrition), decreased absorption of iron (e.g., small bowel disease, gastric bypass), or overt or occult loss of blood. Once the diagnosis of iron deficiency anemia is established, the workup depends on coexisting symptoms, patient's age, and sex.

A. Iron deficiency anemia is defined as hemoglobin <13 g/dL in men and <12 g/dL in nonpregnant women, combined with a ferritin value of <45 ng/mL. Iron deficiency anemia can also be diagnosed at higher ferritin levels, based on increased total iron binding capacity, low serum iron level, and low transferring saturation.

B. The clinical history should be reviewed to evaluate for obvious causes of iron deficiency anemia. Ask about the gastrointestinal (GI) symptoms such as overt bleeding (hematemesis, melena, hematochezia), abdominal pain, and diarrhea. Other symptoms include bleeding from other organ systems (severe hemoptysis, hematuria, epistaxis) and menorrhagia. Strict vegan or vegetarian diet may induce iron deficiency anemia.

C. In patients with overt bleeding or other GI symptoms (e.g., dysphagia, abdominal pain, abnormal imaging of the GI tract), endoscopic workup should proceed based on the most likely site of bleeding.

D. Premenopausal women with abnormal uterine bleeding should be evaluated and treated by gynecology, and treatment with oral iron replacement is reasonable. Hemoglobin improvement is usually observed after 1 month of oral iron replacement. In those who respond to treatment, further workup is not necessary. However, if abnormal uterine bleeding resolves and iron deficiency anemia persists, then further workup should be pursued.

E. The American Gastroenterology Association (AGA) recommends bidirectional endoscopy (esophagogastroduodenoscopy and colonoscopy) for asymptomatic premenopausal women with iron deficiency anemia. However, a conservative approach is also suggested for some patients who would like to defer endoscopy. In these patients, treatment with iron replacement therapy and monitoring the blood count for response is reasonable.

F. In asymptomatic men or postmenopausal women, bidirectional endoscopy should be performed for further evaluation. *Helicobacter pylori* infection and celiac disease are known etiologies for iron deficiency anemia. In patients without prior testing for *H. pylori* or celiac disease, consider obtaining gastric biopsies and small bowel biopsies during the upper endoscopy.

G. If a source of bleeding is identified by endoscopy, then further treatment should address this specific etiology. If bidirectional endoscopy does not reveal a cause of iron deficiency anemia, the AGA recommends treatment with iron replacement therapy and monitoring response to treatment. However, some physicians would proceed directly to small bowel capsule endoscopy for further workup.

H. In patients who do not respond to iron replacement therapy, capsule endoscopy should be performed to assess the small intestines for any etiology of iron deficiency anemia.

I. If a lesion is identified on capsule endoscopy, then further workup depends on the type and location of the lesion. An actively bleeding angiectasia in the jejunum may require push or deep enteroscopy for treatment. A patient with few nonbleeding angioectasias may only require iron replacement therapy and clinical follow-up. A small bowel mass may require endoscopy for biopsy and additional cross-sectional imaging.

J. If capsule endoscopy is normal, most patients would require clinical follow-up and iron replacement therapy alone. In patients with persistent severe iron deficiency anemia, repeat endoscopy or additional imaging tests may be required for further workup.

BIBLIOGRAPHY

1. Ko CW, Siddique SM, Patel A, et al. AGA Clinical practice guidelines on the gastrointestinal evaluation of iron deficiency anemia. *Gastroenterology.* 2020;159(3):1085–1094. https://doi.org/10.1053/j.gastro.2020.06.046.

ALGORITHM 18.1 Flowchart for the workup and management of iron deficiency anemia.

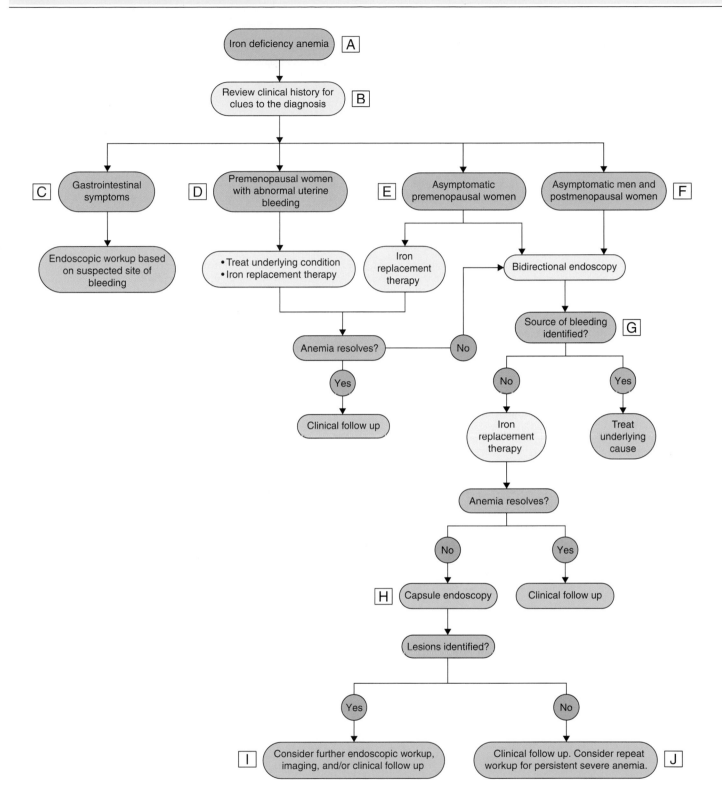

19 | **Foreign Body Ingestion**

Nikrad Shahnavaz

Most cases of foreign body ingestion resolve without serious clinical sequelae. The decision to perform endoscopy and its timing depend on several factors, including presence of symptoms, location, size, shape, and content of the ingested object. The clinical history and two-view plain radiographs (without contrast) are usually sufficient to obtain the necessary information and guide management. Computed tomography (CT) scan is rarely required, but it has higher sensitivity to detect smaller objects and potential complication such as perforation or abscess. Wood, plastic, glass, fish, or chicken bones are not usually seen with plain radiographs.

A. Caustic ingestions in adults usually occur as suicide attempts. Chest x-ray or CT of the neck, chest, and abdomen should be ordered first to rule out perforation and the need for emergent surgery. If perforation is ruled out, upper endoscopy is indicated in 24 to 48 hours after ingestion to grade the degree of injury, establish a prognosis, and guide further treatment. A second endoscopy at 5 days postingestion may help better to predict the prognosis. Refer to Chapter 20 (Caustic Ingestions) for a detailed management algorithm of caustic ingestions.

B. If ingestion of narcotic packets is suspected, then endoscopy is contraindicated due to the risk of package perforation and drug overdose. The patient should be placed on clear liquid diet and monitored with serial radiographs to rule out bowel obstruction, failure to progress, or drug leakage requiring surgical intervention.

C. In patients with complete esophageal obstruction (with drooling and inability to manage oral secretions), emergent endoscopy within 2–6 hours is indicated. If there are sharp-pointed objects or disk batteries in the esophagus, emergent endoscopy is required to reduce the risk of esophageal perforation or necrosis. All other scenarios with foreign body in the esophagus warrant endoscopic removal within 24 hours. Intravenous administration of glucagon 1 mg, while endoscopy is coordinated, could be considered in the setting of food bolus impaction in the esophagus.

D. Most small blunt objects (diameter less than 2.5 cm) which enter the stomach will pass spontaneously. Therefore, asymptomatic patients can be observed and managed conservatively. Endoscopic removal is indicated if objects stay in the stomach or proximal duodenum longer than 3–4 weeks. Sharp-pointed objects, long objects (longer than 5–6 cm), or magnets within endoscopic reach should be removed within 24 hours to reduce the risk of any damage to the stomach. All types of batteries or large blunt objects which stay in the stomach for more than 48 hours need endoscopic removal.

E. The risk of complications such as bleeding or perforation caused by a sharp-pointed object that enters the stomach is as high as 35%. When these objects are beyond the reach of upper endoscopy, they should be monitored closely with daily radiographs to confirm their passage. If the object fails to progress after 72 hours, or if the patient complains of abdominal pain, vomiting, fever, melena, or hematemesis, surgical intervention should be considered.

F. Blunt objects which pass into the distal duodenum can usually exit the gut without any complication. However, they need to be observed weekly with radiographs until they enter the colon. If no progress is witnessed after 1 week, the decision to remove them either with balloon enteroscopy or surgery should be considered based on the patient's condition and local expertise.

BIBLIOGRAPHY

1. Sleisenger and Fordtran's Gastrointestinal and Liver Disease, 11th Edition, 2020.
2. Birk M, Bauerfeind P, Deprez PH, et al. Removal of foreign bodies in the upper gastrointestinal tract in adults: European Society of Gastrointestinal Endoscopy (ESGE) Clinical Guideline. *Endoscopy*. 2016;48(5):489-496.
3. ASGE Standards of Practice Committee Ikenberry SO, Jue TL, Anderson MA, et al. Management of ingested foreign bodies and food impactions. *Gastrointest Endosc*. 2011;73(6):1085-1091.

ALGORITHM 19.1 Flowchart for the workup and management of a patient with foreign body ingestion. *CT*, Computed tomography.

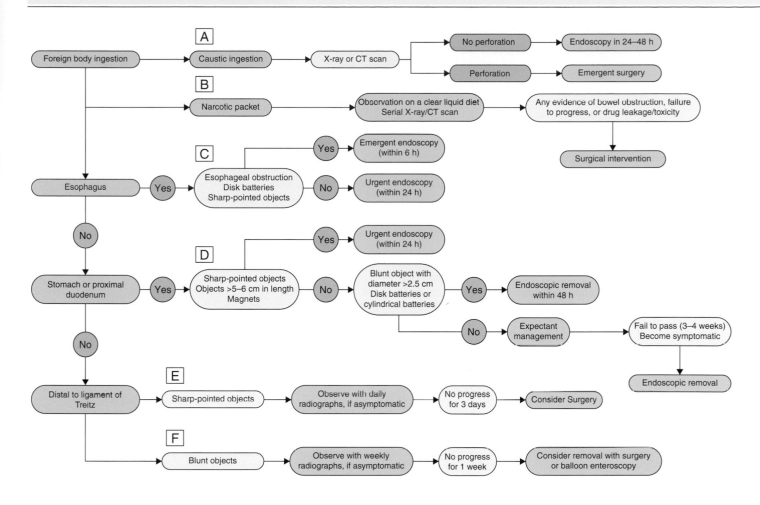

20 Caustic Ingestions

Emad Qayed

Ingestion of caustic substances can occur in the setting of suicide attempts, mental health disorders, alcohol intoxication, and accidental ingestions. The severity of oropharyngeal, esophageal, and upper gastrointestinal injury depends on the pH of the substance, the amount ingested, and its concentration. Alkali is present in household cleaning solutions and drain opening products such as lye. Ingestion of strong alkali (pH >12) can cause severe liquefactive necrosis of the tissue and deep transmural injury, while ingestion of strong acids (pH <2) leads to coagulative necrosis.

A. Patients presenting with acute caustic ingestion should be asked about the type and amount of caustic substance, the presence of laryngeal and respiratory symptoms (hoarseness, stridor, chest pain), and gastrointestinal symptoms (oral pain, dysphagia, odynophagia, hematemesis, abdominal pain). The exam should look for signs of oral injury, cardiopulmonary abnormalities, and abdominal tenderness. Basic laboratory workup includes complete blood count and complete metabolic profile.

B. Presence of laryngeal signs (hoarseness and stridor) or severe respiratory distress requires laryngoscopy and consideration of endotracheal intubation.

C. Chest and abdominal radiographs are useful to examine for signs of perforation (pneumomediastinum, pneumoperitoneum, and pneumothorax, pleural effusion). Computed tomography (CT) scan of the neck, chest, and abdomen should be performed if there is a high suspicion of perforation and/or severe caustic injury to the upper gastrointestinal tract.

D. In patients with confirmed or suspected perforation, intravenous antibiotics should be administered and urgent surgical consultation should be obtained. Esophagogastroduodenoscopy (EGD) should be avoided. The decision to pursue emergent versus delayed operative intervention (e.g., esophagectomy, gastrectomy) depends on the type and extent of perforation and stability of the patient to undergo surgery. Referral to centers with expertise in these types of surgery is appropriate.

E. In asymptomatic patients with a history of accidental, low-volume ingestion of low concentration substance, EGD is not necessary,

and they can be discharged home. EGD should be performed within 24–48 hours in all other patients without confirmed or suspected perforation. EGD provides valuable information about the extent of esophageal, gastric, and duodenal injury and outlines further management.

F. Patients with normal upper endoscopy should be discharged early.

G. Patients with mild mucosal injury (grade I or IIA) should be given a proton pump inhibitor (PPI) and considered for early discharge. Symptomatic patients with more extensive esophagitis or gastritis can be started on oral diet, observed for 24–48 hours, and discharged.

H. Patients with severe mucosal injury (grade IIB or III) should receive PPI, be placed nil per os (NPO) for 24–48 hours, then started on liquid diet and advanced slowly. Consider admission to the intensive care unit for close observation.

I. In patients who are found to have a perforation during endoscopy, intravenous antibiotics should be administered and urgent surgical consultation should be obtained.

J. Clinical follow-up is recommended in patients with extensive mucosal injury, because these patients may develop late complications such as esophageal or pyloric strictures. Treatment requires endoscopic dilation, or surgical therapy in refractory cases. Esophageal cancer can develop years after sustaining a mucosal caustic injury. In those with significant mucosal injury, EGD is recommended every 1–3 years starting 15–20 years after esophageal caustic injury.

BIBLIOGRAPHY

1. De Lusong MAA, Timbol ABG, Tuazon DJS. Management of esophageal caustic injury. *World J Gastrointest Pharmacol Ther.* 2017;8(2):90–98. https://doi.org/10.4292/wjgpt.v8.i2.90.
2. Tosca J, Sánchez A, Sanahuja A, et al. Caustic ingestion: a risk-based algorithm. *Am J Gastroenterol.* 2022;117(10):1593–1604. https://doi.org/10.14309/ajg.0000000000001953.

ALGORITHM 20.1 Flowchart for the workup and management of acute caustic ingestion. *CT*, Computed tomography; *EGD*, esophagogastroduodenoscopy; *IV*, intravenous; *PPI*, proton pump inhibitor; *NPO*, nil per os.

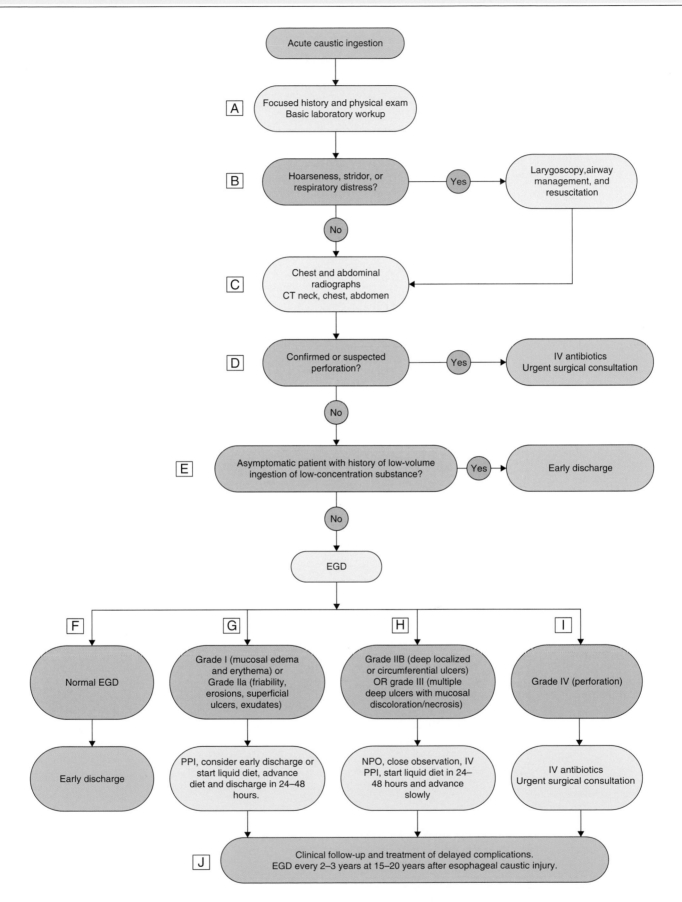

Acute caustic ingestion

A — Focused history and physical exam
Basic laboratory workup

B — Hoarseness, stridor, or respiratory distress? → Yes → Larygoscopy, airway management, and resuscitation

No

C — Chest and abdominal radiographs
CT neck, chest, abdomen

D — Confirmed or suspected perforation? → Yes → IV antibiotics
Urgent surgical consultation

No

E — Asymptomatic patient with history of low-volume ingestion of low-concentration substance? → Yes → Early discharge

No

EGD

F — Normal EGD → Early discharge

G — Grade I (mucosal edema and erythema) or Grade IIa (friability, erosions, superficial ulcers, exudates) → PPI, consider early discharge or start liquid diet, advance diet and discharge in 24–48 hours.

H — Grade IIB (deep localized or circumferential ulcers) OR grade III (multiple deep ulcers with mucosal discoloration/necrosis) → NPO, close observation, IV PPI, start liquid diet in 24–48 hours and advance slowly

I — Grade IV (perforation) → IV antibiotics
Urgent surgical consultation

J — Clinical follow-up and treatment of delayed complications.
EGD every 2–3 years at 15–20 years after esophageal caustic injury.

PART II
Specific Gastrointestinal Disorders

Barrett's Esophagus

Emad Qayed

Barrett's esophagus (BE) refers to the acquired metaplastic condition in which the distal esophageal squamous epithelium changes to columnar (intestinal) epithelium. Further metaplastic changes lead to the development of low-grade dysplasia, high-grade dysplasia, and adenocarcinoma. The histologic diagnosis of BE-related dysplasia should always be confirmed by two expert pathologists

The approach to the diagnosis and management of BE depends on the presence and absence of dysplasia and other esophageal lesions.

A. BE can be diagnosed during an upper endoscopy performed for various indications. Specific screening for BE is recommended in patients with chronic symptoms of gastroesophageal reflux disease (GERD) (heartburn and regurgitation) combined with other risk factors for esophageal adenocarcinoma such as males, age ≥50 years, White individuals, central obesity, current or past history of smoking, and first-degree relative with BE or esophageal adenocarcinoma.

B. The gastroesophageal junction should normally be present at the level of the top of the gastric folds. BE is recognized endoscopically as the extension of the salmon-colored mucosa more than 1 cm above the gastroesophageal junction.

C. The extent of BE should be noted by examining the circumferential extent and maximal extent of salmon-colored mucosa (Prague classification). The BE mucosa should be examined closely for any mucosal lesions, ulcerations, and nodularities. The location of esophageal landmarks and findings should be clearly and accurately documented. Nodules should be biopsied separately with mucosal biopsy or with excisional biopsy using endoscopic mucosal resection (EMR) or endoscopic submucosal dissection (ESD). Biopsies should be obtained from the BE mucosa, with four bites every 2 cm to adequately examine for BE and dysplasia. Patients with confirmed BE should receive proton pump inhibitors (PPIs) to treat underlying GERD.

D. If BE is adequately sampled and there is no dysplasia, then a repeat esophagogastroduodenoscopy (EGD) every 3–5 years is recommended for surveillance. EGD every 5 years is suggested for short-segment nondysplastic BE (<3 cm in length), and every 3 years for long-segment nondysplastic BE (≥3 cm).

E. If histology shows mucosal abnormalities that are indefinite for dysplasia, it is recommended to optimize PPI therapy and repeat EGD within 3–6 months for additional-biopsies.

F. If histology shows low-grade dysplasia that is confirmed by two pathologists, a repeat endoscopy is recommended to confirm the diagnosis within 3–6 months. If low-grade dysplasia is confirmed, then endoscopic ablation with radiofrequency ablation (RFA) or other ablative methods is recommended. Following complete ablation, surveillance is recommended at 1 year and 3 years. An alternative, less preferred approach is endoscopic surveillance for low-grade dysplasia.

G. If histology shows high-grade dysplasia that is confirmed by two pathologists, a repeat endoscopy is recommended to confirm the diagnosis within 3 months. If high-grade dysplasia is confirmed, then endoscopic ablation is recommended. Following complete ablation, surveillance is recommended at 3, 6, and 12 months then annually.

H. The presence of a nodule within BE mucosa should raise suspicion for high-grade dysplasia or early esophageal adenocarcinoma. The nodular lesion should be resected using EMR to allow for adequate histologic examination and staging.

I. If adenocarcinoma is diagnosed based on EMR or ESD specimen, further management depends on the extent of the tumor. Complete endoscopic resection of mucosal adenocarcinoma (T1a) is considered adequate therapy to treat the tumor. This should be followed by endoscopic ablation of BE mucosa.

J. If the EMR specimen shows submucosal adenocarcinoma without high-risk histologic features (>500 μm submucosal invasion, presence of lymphatic invasion), then EMR or ESD is considered adequate therapy, especially if the patient is at high risk for surgery. Patients with T1B tumors with high-risk features should be evaluated for esophagectomy.

BIBLIOGRAPHY

1. Shaheen NJ, Falk GW, Iyer PG, et al. Diagnosis and management of Barrett's ssophagus: an updated ACG guideline. *Am J Gastroenterol*. 2022;117(4):559–587. https://doi.org/10.14309/ajg.0000000000001680.
2. Muthusamy VR, Wani S, Gyawali CP, Komanduri S, CGIT Barrett's Esophagus Consensus Conference Participants. AGA clinical practice update on new technology and innovation for surveillance and screening in Barrett's esophagus: expert review. *Clin Gastroenterol Hepatol*. 2022;20(12):2696–2706.e1. https://doi.org/10.1016/j.cgh.2022.06.003.

ALGORITHM 21.1 Flowchart for the diagnosis and management of Barrett's esophagus. *BE*, Barrett's esophagus; *EGD*, esophagogastroduodenoscopy; *PPI*, proton pump inhibitor.

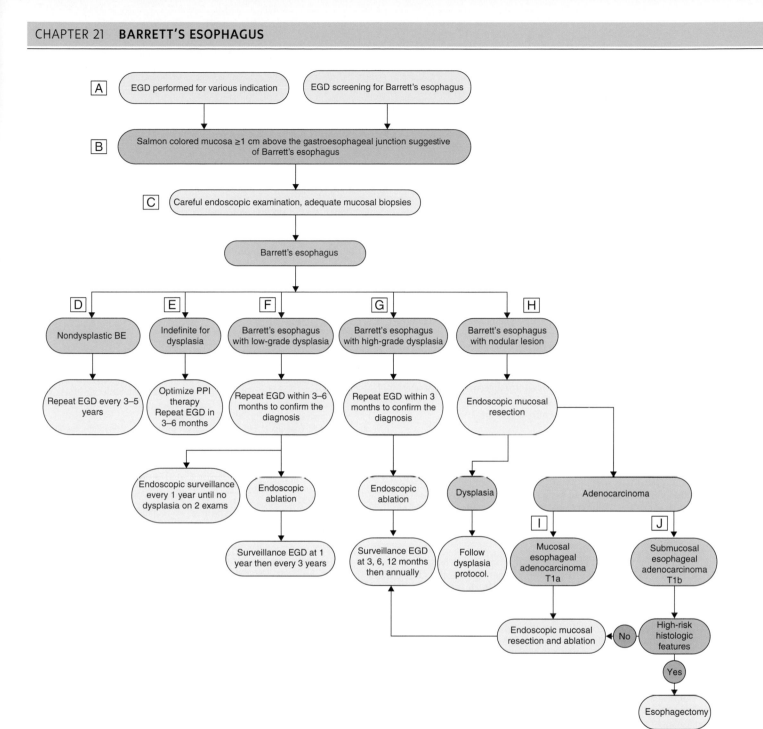

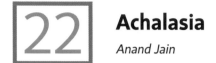

Achalasia

Anand Jain

Treatment of achalasia is aimed at improving opening of the lower esophageal sphincter (LES) muscle. This is accomplished by permanent disruption of the muscle fibers by one of two procedures: myotomy or pneumatic dilation. Both procedures have an 80% or higher efficacy in reducing dysphagia severity. Myotomy can be performed via two approaches: (1) a laparoscopic surgical approach termed a Heller myotomy, typically performed laparoscopically (LHM), and (2) per oral endoscopic myotomy (POEM), which is an incisionless approach performed during endoscopy.

A. An important consideration in choice of therapy for achalasia is the anatomy of the esophagus. In achalasia, there is esophageal wall remodeling due to hydrostatic forces related to bolus retention and LES obstruction. As such, some achalasia patients can have a severely dilated esophagus diffusely (termed megaesophagus), or more focal dilatation in the form of diverticula proximal to areas of obstruction or spasm. In these circumstances, LES opening alone is unlikely to improve bolus flow dynamics, and consideration for esophagectomy, or Heller myotomy with straightening of the esophagus and/or diverticulectomy, may be necessary. For this reason, patients should be referred to an esophageal center if significant anatomical deformity is present.

B. There are clinical scenarios in which myotomy or pneumatic dilation may not be safe, such as in elderly patients, patients on anticoagulation or antiplatelet therapy that would be high risk to discontinue periprocedurally, or patients in whom anesthesia, and particularly endotracheal intubation, carries a high risk. In these patients, a trial of botulinum toxin injection to the LES (100 units injected during esophagogastroduodenoscopy [EGD]) and a trial of pharmacologic smooth muscle relaxants (nitrates, calcium channel blockers, sildenafil) are reasonable options.

C. In addition to the difference in approach, a key difference between LHM and POEM is that Heller myotomy generally includes an antireflux procedure performed at the same time which is usually in the form of a partial (Dor or Toupet) fundoplication. Rates of pathologic reflux after POEM are higher than after LHM and might be as high as 40%. Pneumatic dilation entails circumferential stretch of the LES via a rigid balloon with diameter sizes 30 or 35 mm (although 40-mm balloons exist, we do not recommend use given the higher rates of perforation with this size). The key factor that should influence the choice of therapy is the manometric achalasia subtype. Type 2 achalasia has the best response to all therapies; type 1 achalasia has less response to pneumatic dilation; and type 3 achalasia generally warrants a long myotomy which is often technically the easiest to perform with POEM.

D. Achalasia is a chronic disease, and LES muscle dysfunction recurs in a sizable proportion (~20% recurrence rate at 5 years if combining all interventions) after a successful opening procedure. Ongoing esophageal remodeling can also occur which can cause esophageal dilatation and advanced deformity. Also, although relatively rare, there is the possibility that LES dysfunction could convert to a spastic phenotype with esophageal body dysfunction spasm, even after an opening procedure for the LES. A unique consideration for patients who undergo LHM with a fundoplication is that the fundoplication can herniate or slip and cause a functional obstruction at the esophago-gastric junction (EGJ). For all of the earlier reasons, patients with achalasia should be assessed periodically after the initial treatment intervention. Our recommendation is to perform a symptom assessment and timed barium esophagogram (TBE) 3 months after the intervention.

E. Patients with a good outcome and durable improvement in dysphagia should still incur a symptom assessment every 6 months, and a TBE every 2 years.

F. Patients who do not respond to the initial opening procedure or have recurrent dysphagia that develops after an initially successful treatment procedure should be referred to an esophageal center such that a complete workup with state-of-the-art diagnostics (EGD, high-resolution manometry, endoluminal functional lumen imaging probe, TBE) can be performed to direct management.

BIBLIOGRAPHY

1. Spiess AE, Kahrilas PJ. Treating achalasia: from whalebone to laparoscope. *JAMA.* 1998;280:638-642.
2. Yaghoobi M, Mayrand S, Martel M, et al. Laparoscopic Heller's myotomy versus pneumatic dilation in the treatment of idiopathic achalasia: a meta-analysis of randomized, controlled trials. *Gastrointest Endosc.* 2013;78:468-475.
3. Schlottmann F, Luckett DJ, Fine J, et al. Laparoscopic Heller myotomy versus peroral endoscopic myotomy (POEM) for achalasia: a systematic review and meta-analysis. *Ann Surg.* 2018;267:451-460.
4. Ponds FA, Fockens P, Lei A, et al. Effect of peroral endoscopic myotomy vs pneumatic dilation on symptom severity and treatment outcomes among treatment-naive patients with achalasia: a randomized clinical trial. *JAMA.* 2019;322:134-144.
5. Pandolfino JE, Kwiatek MA, Nealis T, et al. Achalasia: a new clinically relevant classification by high-resolution manometry. *Gastroenterology.* 2008;135:1526-1533.
6. Yadlapati R, Kahrilas PJ, Fox MR, et al. Esophageal motility disorders on high-resolution manometry: Chicago Classification Version 4.0((c)). *Neurogastroenterol Motil.* 2021;33:e14058.
7. Pratap N, Kalapala R, Darisetty S, et al. Achalasia cardia subtyping by high-resolution manometry predicts the therapeutic outcome of pneumatic balloon dilatation. *J Neurogastroenterol Motil.* 2011;17:48-53.
8. Farhoomand K, Connor JT, Richter JE, et al. Predictors of outcome of pneumatic dilation in achalasia. *Clin Gastroenterol Hepatol.* 2004;2:389-394.
9. Salvador R, Costantini M, Zaninotto G, et al. The preoperative manometric pattern predicts the outcome of surgical treatment for esophageal achalasia. *J Gastrointest Surg.* 2010;14:1635-1645.
10. Rohof WO, Salvador R, Annese V, et al. Outcomes of treatment for achalasia depend on manometric subtype. *Gastroenterology.* 2013;144:718-725. quiz e13-4.
11. Kumbhari V, Tieu AH, Onimaru M, et al. Peroral endoscopic myotomy (POEM) vs laparoscopic Heller myotomy (LHM) for the treatment of type III achalasia in 75 patients: a multicenter comparative study. *Endosc Int Open.* 2015;3:E195-E201.
12. Jain AS, Carlson DA, Triggs J, et al. Esophagogastric junction distensibility on functional lumen imaging probe topography predicts treatment response in achalasia—anatomy matters! *Am J Gastroenterol.* 2019;114:1455-1463.
13. Birgisson S, Richter JE. Long-term outcome of botulinum toxin in the treatment of achalasia. *Gastroenterology.* 1996;111:1162-1163.
14. Bortolotti M, Mari C, Lopilato C, et al. Effects of sildenafil on esophageal motility of patients with idiopathic achalasia. *Gastroenterology.* 2000;118:253-257.
15. West RL, Hirsch DP, Bartelsman JF, et al. Long term results of pneumatic dilation in achalasia followed for more than 5 years. *Am J Gastroenterol.* 2002;97:1346-1351.
16. Vela MF, Richter JE, Khandwala F, et al. The long-term efficacy of pneumatic dilatation and Heller myotomy for the treatment of achalasia. *Clin Gastroenterol Hepatol.* 2006;4:580-587.
17. Jeansonne LO, White BC, Pilger KE, et al. Ten-year follow-up of laparoscopic Heller myotomy for achalasia shows durability. *Surg Endosc.* 2007;21:1498-1502.

ALGORITHM 22.1 Management of achalasia. *EndoFLIP,* Endoluminal functional lumen imaging probe; *HRM,* high-resolution manometry; *LES,* lower esophageal sphincter; *LHM,* laparoscopic Heller myotomy; *POEM,* per oral endoscopic myotomy; *TBE,* timed barium esophagogram.

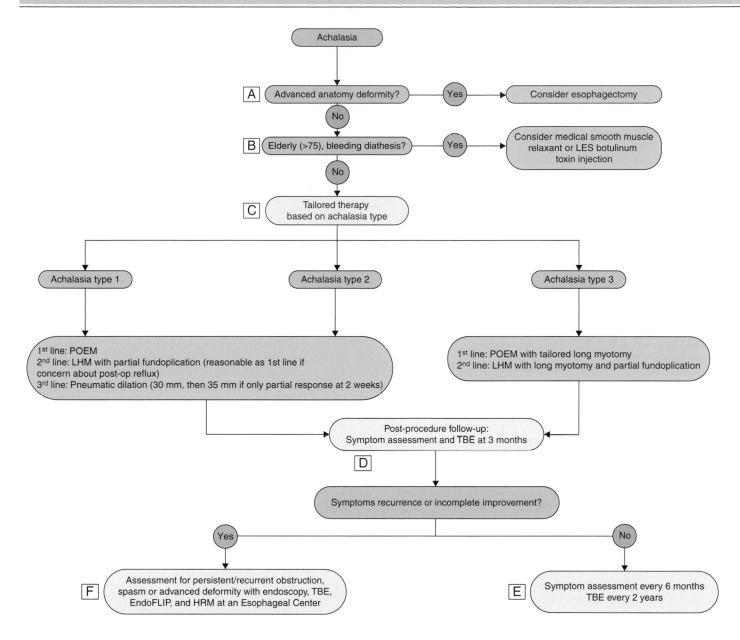

Eosinophilic Esophagitis

Emad Qayed

Eosinophilic esophagitis (EoE) is a chronic immune-mediated inflammatory disorder of the esophagus characterized clinically by symptoms of esophageal dysfunction, and histologically by mucosal eosinophilic infiltration.

A. Patients usually present with persistent symptoms of dysphagia, chest pain, heartburn, and/or regurgitation. They may experience episodes of food impaction requiring urgent endoscopy.

B. An esophagogastroduodenoscopy (EGD) is the test of choice for persistent esophageal symptoms, as it can diagnose a myriad of esophageal pathology (e.g., strictures, peptic esophagitis, and malignancy). Supportive endoscopic findings of EoE include esophageal rings, white exudates, longitudinal furrows, edema, narrow-caliber esophagus, and esophageal mucosal fragility manifested by ulcerations induced by passage of the endoscope (crêpe-paper esophagus). Regardless of endoscopic findings, biopsies should be obtained from the proximal and distal esophagus to examine for esophageal eosinophilic infiltration. In patients with a suspicion of gastroesophageal reflux disease (GERD), separating these biopsies into proximal and distal jars may aid in differentiating GERD from EoE. GERD may induce mild eosinophilia in the distal esophagus, while EoE leads to more significant eosinophilia in both the distal and proximal esophagus. In patients with food impaction, it is recommended that biopsies are obtained during the same endoscopy session, to avoid the need for repeat endoscopy and biopsy. It is also preferable that biopsies are obtained off proton pump inhibitors (PPIs) because these drugs can treat esophageal eosinophilia and therefore mask the diagnosis of EoE. In patients with compatible symptoms, gastric and duodenal biopsies should be obtained to rule out eosinophilic gastroenteritis.

C. If histology shows ≥15 eosinophils per high-power field (HPF), other causes of esophageal eosinophilia should be considered, most importantly GERD. It is appropriate to perform an esophageal pH study to evaluate for GERD if there is a high clinical suspicion. Other less common causes of esophageal eosinophilia are eosinophilic gastroenteritis, Crohn's disease, achalasia, vasculitis, drug hypersensitivity response, and parasitic infections. Previously, the diagnosis of EoE required a treatment trial with PPI to rule out an entity called "PPI responsive esophageal eosinophilia" (PPI-REE). This is no longer required because PPI-REE is considered a subset of EoE.

D. If histology does not show esophageal eosinophilia, consider other causes of esophageal symptoms and treat accordingly (e.g., esophageal manometry, esophageal pH testing).

E. First-line treatment options for EoE include PPI, topical swallowed steroids (fluticasone, viscous budesonide), and dietary therapy (elimination diet). Dupilumab is a human monoclonal IgG4 antibody that inhibits interleukin-4 (IL-4) and IL-13 and is approved for the treatment of EoE. In selected patients with high-grade esophageal stricture, dilation can be attempted before medical therapy to provide symptom relief. However, most patients should receive medical therapy to treat the underlying inflammation before attempting esophageal dilation.

F. If clinical response is achieved, then long-term maintenance therapy is recommended to avoid relapse. Some physicians repeat the endoscopy to biopsy the esophagus and confirm endoscopic response to treatment by monitoring the improvement in endoscopic and histologic manifestations of EoE.

G. In patients who do not respond to a particular treatment, an alternative medical therapy should be prescribed. Repeat endoscopy and biopsy are reasonable to assess endoscopic and histologic response to treatment. Esophageal dilation should be performed if there are significant esophageal strictures.

BIBLIOGRAPHY

1. Aceves SS, Alexander JA, Baron TH, et al. Endoscopic approach to eosinophilic esophagitis: American Society for Gastrointestinal Endoscopy Consensus Conference. *Gastrointest Endosc.* 2022;96(4):576–592.e1. https://doi.org/10.1016/j.gie.2022.05.013.
2. Dellon ES, Liacouras CA, Molina-Infante J, et al. Updated international consensus diagnostic criteria for eosinophilic esophagitis: proceedings of the AGREE conference. *Gastroenterology.* 2018;155(4):1022–1033.e10. https://doi.org/10.1053/j.gastro.2018.07.009.

ALGORITHM 23.1 Flowchart for the workup and diagnosis of eosinophilic esophagitis. *EGD*, Esophagogastroduodenoscopy; *PPI*, proton pump inhibitor.

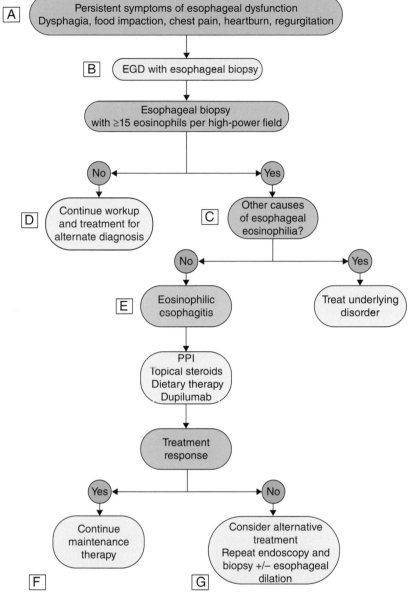

Esophageal Motility Disorders

Anand Jain

Esophageal motility disorders are complex and heterogenous clinical conditions that are identified as distinct patterns on high-resolution manometry (HRM). Chicago Classification version 4.0 (CC v4.0) defines six disorders: (1) achalasia (note that there are three distinct subtypes), (2) esophagogastric junction outflow obstruction (EGJOO), (3) absent contractility, (4) ineffective esophageal motility (IEM), (5) distal esophageal spasm, and (6) hypercontractile esophagus.

A. The typical indication for HRM is nonobstructive dysphagia. HRM is also indicated for noncardiac chest pain and in the case of suspected gastroesophageal reflux disease (GERD) in order to measure the gastroesophageal junction location for pH catheter placement, or where there is intent to consider antireflux surgery (ARS). Management of each pattern should be guided by the scenario under which it is diagnosed.

B. Achalasia is the most severe motility disorder and carries the risk of long-term esophageal remodeling, significant dysphagia, and aspiration. As such, regardless of whether it is detected in the presence of obstructive symptoms (dysphagia and/or noncardiac chest pain) or GERD symptoms, it should be treated with a definitive intervention to open the lower esophageal sphincter (LES) (pneumatic dilation or myotomy), which should be guided by the achalasia subtype.

C. EGJOO is a common manometric diagnosis, with many questions to be answered regarding pathogenesis and clinical course. EGJOO detected in the setting of obstructive symptoms should be treated. Given the lack of systematic clinical trial data in EGJOO to guide therapy, our approach is to perform an LES botulinum toxin (Botox) injection as initial therapy, followed by pneumatic dilation, and lastly myotomy, for refractory cases.

D. The optimal management of EGJOO detected in the setting of GERD symptoms or on preoperative ARS testing is unclear. Our approach is to escalate proton pump inhibitor (PPI) therapy and to repeat esophageal function testing in 6 months. If the EGJOO persists and the severity of GERD symptoms warrants ARS, this author would consider a partial fundoplication ± myotomy in lieu of a complete fundoplication.

E. Absent contractility or IEM—disorders of hypomotility typically contribute to reflux burden due to poor acid clearance, or slow transit dysphagia. Thus, these findings should prompt aggressive reflux control. When encountered on pre-ARS testing, these findings should direct the surgical approach toward a partial fundoplication in lieu of a full Nissen fundoplication.

F. If absent contractility or IEM is detected in a patient with dysphagia, then referral to speech and swallow therapist is appropriate for assessment of bolus transit with various food consistencies and trials of dietary modification strategies.

G. Distal esophageal spasm and hypercontractile esophagus are additional patterns that could cause esophageal obstruction and/or chest pain. In the presence of these symptoms, these patterns should prompt treatment with pharmacologic smooth muscle relaxants (nitrates, calcium channel blockers, or sildenafil).

H. When distal esophageal spasm or hypercontractile esophagus is detected during evaluation for GERD symptoms, we recommend escalation of PPI for 6 months followed by repeat HRM. If the pattern persists and the severity of GERD warrants ARS, this author would consider a partial fundoplication in lieu of a complete fundoplication.

BIBLIOGRAPHY

1. Yadlapati R, Kahrilas PJ, Fox MR, et al. Esophageal motility disorders on high-resolution manometry: Chicago Classification Version 4.0((c)). *Neurogastroenterol Motil.* 2021;33:e14058.
2. Zaninotto G, Bennett C, Boeckxstaens G, et al. The 2018 ISDE achalasia guidelines. *Dis Esophagus.* 2018:31.
3. Pandolfino JE, Gawron AJ. Achalasia: a systematic review. *JAMA.* 2015;313:1841-1852.
4. Kahrilas PJ, Boeckxstaens G. The spectrum of achalasia: lessons from studies of pathophysiology and high-resolution manometry. *Gastroenterology.* 2013;145:954-965.
5. Rohof WO, Salvador R, Annese V, et al. Outcomes of treatment for achalasia depend on manometric subtype. *Gastroenterology.* 2013;144:718-725. quiz e13-4.
6. Perez-Fernandez MT, Santander C, Marinero A, et al. Characterization and follow-up of esophagogastric junction outflow obstruction detected by high resolution manometry. *Neurogastroenterol Motil.* 2016;28:116-126.
7. Furuzawa-Carballeda J, Coss-Adame E, Romero-Hernandez F, et al. Esophagogastric junction outflow obstruction: characterization of a new entity? Clinical, manometric, and neuroimmunological description. *Neurogastroenterol Motil.* 2020;32:e13867.
8. Garbarino S, von Isenburg M, Fisher DA, et al. Management of functional esophagogastric junction outflow obstruction: a systematic review. *J Clin Gastroenterol.* 2020;54:35-42.
9. Kovacs B, Masuda T, Bremner RM, et al. Clinical spectrum and presentation of patients with absent contractility. *Ann Gastroenterol.* 2021;34:331-336.
10. Gyawali CP, Zerbib F, Bhatia S, et al. Chicago Classification update (V4.0): technical review on diagnostic criteria for ineffective esophageal motility and absent contractility. *Neurogastroenterol Motil.* 2021;33:e14134.
11. Gyawali CP, Sifrim D, Carlson DA, et al. Ineffective esophageal motility: concepts, future directions, and conclusions from the Stanford 2018 Symposium. *Neurogastroenterol Motil.* 2019;31:e13584.
12. Philonenko S, Roman S, Zerbib F, et al. Jackhammer esophagus: clinical presentation, manometric diagnosis, and therapeutic results—results from a multicenter French cohort. *Neurogastroenterol Motil.* 2020;32:e13918.
13. de Bortoli N, Gyawali PC, Roman S, et al. Hypercontractile esophagus from pathophysiology to management: proceedings of the Pisa Symposium. *Am J Gastroenterol.* 2021;116:263-273.
14. Gorti H, Samo S, Shahnavaz N, et al. Distal esophageal spasm: update on diagnosis and management in the era of high-resolution manometry. *World J Clin Cases.* 2020;8:1026-1032.

ALGORITHM 24.1 Management of esophageal motility disorders based on Chicago Classification version 4.0 (CC v4.0). *ARS,* Antireflux surgery; *DES,* distal esophageal spasm; *EGJOO,* esophagogastric junction outflow obstruction; *GERD,* gastroesophageal reflux disease; *HRM,* high-resolution manometry; *IEM,* ineffective esophageal motility; *LES,* lower esophageal sphincter; *PPI,* proton pump inhibitor.

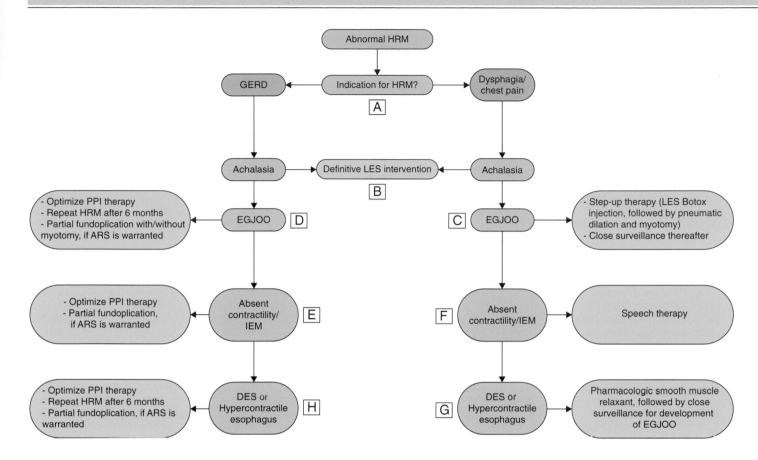

25 *Helicobacter pylori* Infection

Jason M. Brown

Helicobacter pylori is a spiral-shaped, Gram-negative bacterium that lives in the gastric mucous layer. It is generally acknowledged as one of the most common bacterial infections in humans. *H. pylori* infection is typically chronic and acquired in childhood, although variations exist due to demographics and socioeconomic factors. *H. pylori* is strongly associated with the higher rates of gastric cancer, and eradication of *H. pylori* decreases cancer risk. The World Health Organization has recognized *H. pylori* as a class 1 carcinogen, making detection and eradication (with confirmation of eradication) an important and critical clinical task.

A. There are many indications for *H. pylori* testing:
- Established indications
  - Uninvestigated dyspepsia
  - Functional dyspepsia, if not previously tested for *H. pylori*
  - Active peptic ulcer disease
  - Confirmed history of peptic ulcer disease without confirmed prior therapy or eradication testing
  - Low-grade gastric mucosa-associated lymphoid tissue (MALT) lymphoma
  - In patients who have undergone resection of early gastric cancer
  - Long-term nonsteroidal antiinflammatory drug (NSAID) use
- Controversial indications (testing can be considered on an individual basis)
  - Patients taking low-dose aspirin
  - Unexplained iron deficiency anemia
  - Idiopathic thrombocytopenic purpura

B. Patients with symptoms of dyspepsia who are over the age of 60 years or with alarm features should undergo upper endoscopy and biopsy. Alarm features include:
- Dysphagia
- Unexplained weight loss
- Unexplained anemia
- Persistent vomiting
- Abnormal imaging findings of the esophagus, stomach, or the proximal duodenum

C. An esophagogastroduodenoscopy (EGD) and biopsy are performed using the Sydney protocol. This five-biopsy protocol targets the antrum and body along the greater curve, the antrum and body along the lesser curve, and the incisura.

D. Noninvasive diagnostic testing is optimal for patients without alarm features. Urea breath testing and stool antigen testing are the two most commonly used tests for active infection. Both have comparable and acceptable sensitivity and specificity. Of note, proton pump inhibitors (PPIs) should be held for 1–2 weeks prior to any test for *H. pylori* to maximize the sensitivity of the test.

E. Patients with positive stool antigen test, urea breath test, or mucosal biopsy should be treated for *H. pylori*. Testing during an active bleeding episode lowers the sensitivity for infection. Therefore, if a test is negative, consider repeat testing after the acute bleeding episode resolved.

F. The preferred first-line *H. pylori* treatment regimen is the traditional bismuth quadruple therapy (PPI + bismuth + metronidazole + tetracycline) for 14 days. Other potential treatment regimens to consider are as follows:
- Quadruple therapy options
  - PPI + amoxicillin + clarithromycin + metronidazole
- Triple therapy options
  - PPI + amoxicillin + clarithromycin
  - PPI + metronidazole + clarithromycin

G. Posttreatment eradication testing is critical and should be offered to any patient undergoing *H. pylori* therapy. Noninvasive testing for active infection, particularly stool antigen testing, is the test of choice, although this can be made on a case-by-case basis depending on the healthcare system and individual patient scenarios. Testing is recommended 4 weeks post completion of treatment; PPI should be held for 1–2 weeks.

H. If *H. pylori* eradication failed with first-line therapy, a salvage therapy is recommended. All salvage regimens' recommended length is 14 days, except for the rifabutin-containing option, which is 10 days. If the traditional bismuth quadruple therapy (PPI + bismuth + metronidazole + tetracycline) was not given first line, this should be given as a salvage regimen if there are no contraindications to its use. Other potential salvage regimens are considered depending on local antibiotics resistance patterns, and the presence of penicillin allergy.
- PPI + amoxicillin + levofloxacin
- PPI + amoxicillin + rifabutin
- Other bismuth quadruple therapy
  - PPI + Bismuth + levofloxacin + metronidazole
  - PPI + Bismuth + levofloxacin + tetracycline
  - PPI + Bismuth + levofloxacin + amoxicillin
  - PPI + Bismuth + clarithromycin + tetracycline

I. If salvage treatment does not eradicate *H. pylori*, then antibiotic sensitivity testing, if available, should be performed to guide further therapy. Antibiotic sensitivity is assessed using culture-based testing or molecular-based sensitivity testing. Options for subsequent salvage therapy include:
- Retreatment with traditional bismuth quadruple therapy (PPI + bismuth + metronidazole + tetracycline)
- PPI + amoxicillin + rifabutin
- PPI + Bismuth + levofloxacin + metronidazole
- PPI + Bismuth + levofloxacin + tetracycline

In elderly patients without peptic ulcer, gastric atrophy, or intestinal metaplasia, consider not treating *H. pylori* after considering the benefits of eradication versus the risks of repeated antibiotic therapy.

BIBLIOGRAPHY

1. Shah SC, Iyer PG, Moss SF. AGA clinical practice update on the management of refractory *Helicobacter pylori* infection: expert review. *Gastroenterology.* 2021;160(5):1831–1841. https://doi.org/10.1053/j.gastro.2020.11.059.

ALGORITHM 25.1 Flowchart for the diagnosis and treatment of *Helicobacter pylori* infection. *EGD,* Esophagogastroduodenoscopy.

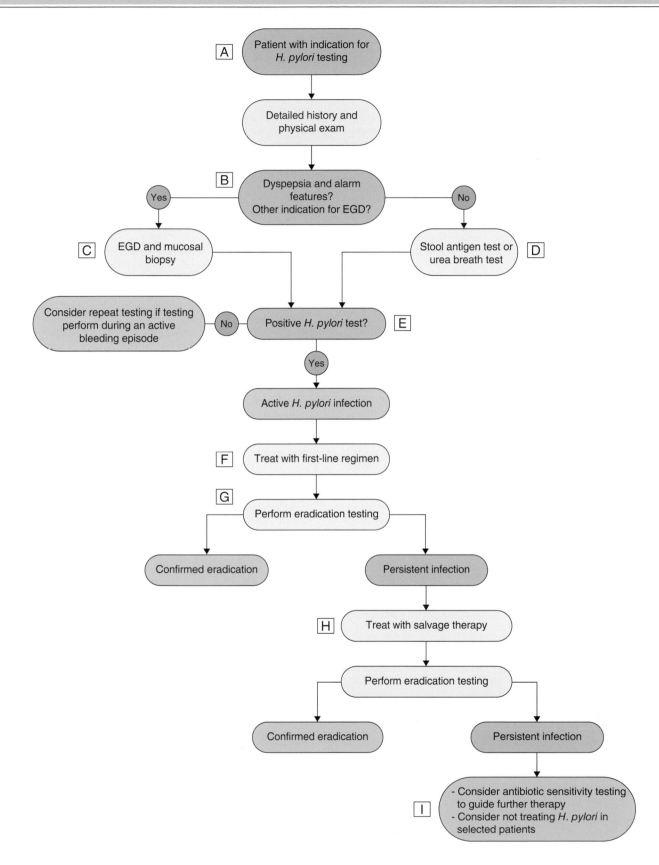

A — Patient with indication for *H. pylori* testing

Detailed history and physical exam

B — Dyspepsia and alarm features? Other indication for EGD?

Yes

No

C — EGD and mucosal biopsy

D — Stool antigen test or urea breath test

Consider repeat testing if testing perform during an active bleeding episode

No

E — Positive *H. pylori* test?

Yes

Active *H. pylori* infection

F — Treat with first-line regimen

G — Perform eradication testing

Confirmed eradication

Persistent infection

H — Treat with salvage therapy

Perform eradication testing

Confirmed eradication

Persistent infection

I —
- Consider antibiotic sensitivity testing to guide further therapy
- Consider not treating *H. pylori* in selected patients

Gastroparesis

Nikrad Shahnavaz

Gastroparesis is motility disorder of the stomach characterized by typical symptoms and objective documentation of delayed gastric emptying of solid food in the absence of mechanical obstruction. The typical symptoms of gastroparesis include chronic nausea, vomiting, bloating, postprandial fullness, and upper abdominal pain. Moreover, refractory gastroesophageal reflux disease (GERD) should trigger workup for gastroparesis.

A. Mechanical obstruction from stricture, ulceration, or tumor can mimic gastroparesis and should be excluded by studies such as endoscopy and/or upper gastrointestinal (GI) contrast studies.

B. Narcotics affect both gastric motility and pyloric function resulting in delay of the gastric emptying. If the patient is on opioids, it should be stopped at least 48 hours prior to gastric emptying study. Other medications that can potentially delay gastric emptying (e.g., anticholinergics, glucagon-like peptide-1 and amylin analogs) should also be discontinued before the test.

C. Scintigraphic gastric emptying of solids over 4 hours is the standard for the diagnosis of gastroparesis. Gastroparesis severity can be categorized based on the extent of gastric emptying delay into mild (10%–15% retention at 4 hours), moderate (15%–35% retention), and severe (>35% retention). Other studies to assess the gastric emptying such as wireless capsule motility testing and ^{13}C spirulina breath testing are acceptable alternatives when available. The presence of food in the stomach at the time of endoscopy is *not* sufficient to make the diagnosis of gastroparesis.

D. Motility disorders of small intestines, colon, or rectal evacuation are commonly seen in patients with gastroparesis. If symptoms suggest, these conditions should be excluded using wireless capsule motility or pan-GI scintigraphy studies.

E. After gastroparesis is diagnosed, the patient should be screened for potential causes such as diabetes mellitus, thyroid diseases, neurological disorders (Parkinson disease), and autoimmune disorders. Marked hyperglycemia (glucose levels above 200 mg/dL) can acutely delay the gastric emptying.

F. The first line of treatment for patients with gastroparesis is dietary modifications, particularly focusing on consumption of frequent small nutrient meals that are low in fat and soluble fiber. Homogenized or liquid food is better tolerated, if the patient cannot tolerate solid food. Consultation with a registered dietician is recommended.

G. Metoclopramide is currently the only Food and Drug Administration (FDA)–approved drug for gastroparesis in the United States. Therefore, it is the first-line pharmacological therapy. Although the risk of tardive dyskinesia (TD) is estimated to be less than 1%, it should be discussed with patients before the initiation of the drug. Patients should be instructed to stop the drug immediately if they develop any side effects including involuntary movements. The risk of TD is higher in elderly women, patients with diabetes or chronic liver or kidney disease, and patients who take antipsychotics.

H. In patients who cannot tolerate metoclopramide or show no clinical response, other prokinetics, including domperidone (under a special FDA program and with electrocardiogram [EKG] monitoring for QT prolongation), prucalopride, or short-term macrolides (erythromycin, clarithromycin, and azithromycin), should be considered. Use of antiemetics, as needed, is recommended to improve associated nausea and vomiting, although they do not affect gastric emptying. For gastroparesis with associated abdominal pain, neuromodulators such as tricyclic antidepressants should be considered.

I. When oral intake is insufficient (weight loss of 10% or more over 3 to 6 months) with repeated hospitalizations for refractory symptoms despite dietary modifications and pharmacological therapy, enteral nutrition by direct jejunostomy tube or gastrojejunostomy tube feeding is strongly recommended. In rare cases, parenteral nutrition is needed.

J. In selected refractory cases of gastroparesis with severe symptoms and severe delay in gastric emptying, gastric electric stimulation (GES), gastric peroral endoscopic myotomy (G-POEM), and laparoscopic pyloroplasty are reasonable treatment options, if performed at a GI motility center of excellence. Intrapyloric injection of botulinum toxin is not recommended because randomized controlled trials have not demonstrated clinical benefit over placebo.

BIBLIOGRAPHY

1. Camilleri M, Kuo B, Nguyen L, Vaughn VM, Petrey J, Greer K, Yadlapati R, Abell TL. ACG clinical guideline: gastroparesis. *Am J Gastroenterol.* 2022;117(8):1197-1220.
2. Lacy BE, Tack J, Gyawali CP. AGA Clinical practice update on management of medically refractory gastroparesis: expert review. *Clin Gastroenterol Hepatol.* 2022;20(3):491-500.
3. Camilleri M, Parkman HP, Shafi MA, Abell TL, Gerson L. American College of Gastroenterology. Clinical guideline: management of gastroparesis. *Am J Gastroenterol.* 2013;108(1):18-37.
4. Sleisenger and Fordtran's Gastrointestinal and Liver Disease, 11th Edition, 2020.

ALGORITHM 26.1 Flowchart for the diagnosis and management of gastroparesis. *GI*, Gastrointestinal; *G-POEM*, gastric per oral endoscopic myotomy.

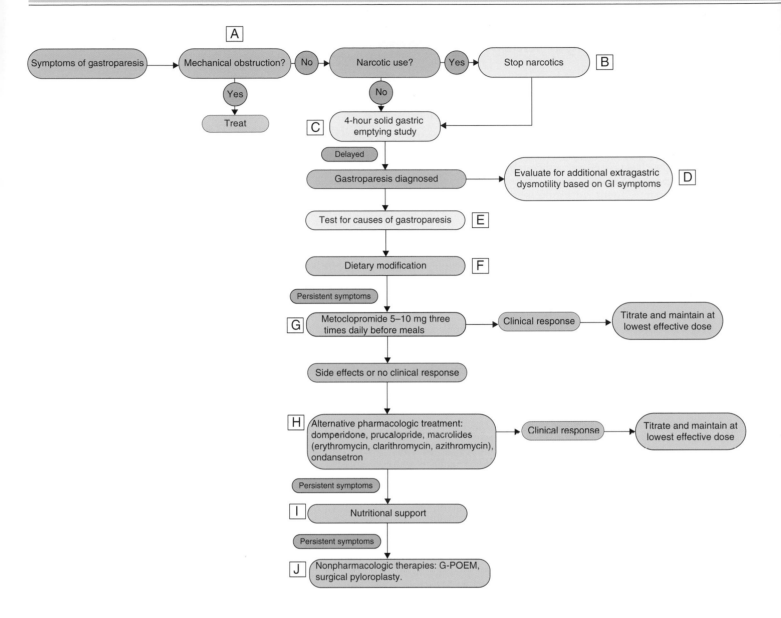

A   Symptoms of gastroparesis → Mechanical obstruction? → No → Narcotic use? → Yes → Stop narcotics   B

Mechanical obstruction? → Yes → Treat

Narcotic use? → No

C   4-hour solid gastric emptying study

Delayed

Gastroparesis diagnosed → Evaluate for additional extragastric dysmotility based on GI symptoms   D

Test for causes of gastroparesis   E

Dietary modification   F

Persistent symptoms

G   Metoclopromide 5–10 mg three times daily before meals → Clinical response → Titrate and maintain at lowest effective dose

Side effects or no clinical response

H   Alternative pharmacologic treatment: domperidone, prucalopride, macrolides (erythromycin, clarithromycin, azithromycin), ondansetron → Clinical response → Titrate and maintain at lowest effective dose

Persistent symptoms

I   Nutritional support

Persistent symptoms

J   Nonpharmacologic therapies: G-POEM, surgical pyloroplasty.

27 Zollinger-Ellison Syndrome

Emad Qayed

Hypergastrinemia is generally categorized into two main categories:

(1) Appropriate hypergastrinemia due to decreased gastric acid production. Examples include gastric acid suppression by histamine (H2) receptor blockers or proton pump inhibitors (PPIs), chronic atrophic gastritis, *Helicobacter pylori* gastritis, and vagotomy without antrectomy. Chronic kidney disease leads to fasting hypergastrinemia due to reduced gastrin clearance.

(2) Inappropriate hypergastrinemia in the setting of normal or increased gastric acid production. Examples are Zollinger-Ellison syndrome (ZES), retained antrum syndrome, and antral G cell hyperplasia. Gastrin stimulates the parietal and pepsin cells (leading to increased gastric acidity), stimulates gastric mucosal blood flow, and has a trophic effect on the gastric and duodenal mucosa.

ZES is caused by excessive gastric acid secretion due to ectopic secretion of gastrin by a neuroendocrine tumor (gastrinoma). This syndrome was first described in 1955 by Zollinger and Ellison in two patients who had extreme acid hypersecretion and severe peptic ulcer disease in the proximal jejunum, caused by a non-beta cell islet tumor of the pancreas. ZES presents with abdominal pain, diarrhea, heartburn, nausea, and vomiting. Patients can develop severe gastroesophageal reflux disease (GERD) and recurrent peptic ulcer disease, with some ulcers in unusual sites such as the distal duodenum and the jejunum. Patients usually present in their fifth or sixth decade of life, and the majority have had symptoms for several years before a diagnosis is made. One in four patients with ZES has multiple endocrine neoplasia, type 1 (MEN 1), which includes hyperparathyroidism, pancreatic endocrine tumor, and pituitary tumor. In general, the diagnosis of ZES relies on the demonstration of inappropriate gastric acid secretion in the presence of hypergastrinemia. Once ZES is diagnosed, further testing is aimed at findings the primary tumor (gastrinoma) using cross-sectional imaging, endoscopic ultrasound, Octreoscan, and other somatostatin imaging studies (e.g., gallium-68 positron emission tomography [PET]).

A. The clinical suspicion of ZES should prompt measurement of fasting serum gastrin (FSG). Fasting hypergastrinemia is found in 97%–99% of patients with ZES. If FSG is not elevated, the chances of ZES are very low (<1%) and most patients are considered not to have ZES. If there is a strong clinical suspicion, some physicians perform the secretin stimulation test for further workup.

B. Patients with elevated FSG should repeat FSG testing off any acid suppression therapy (off PPI for 1 week and H2 receptor blockers for 2 days). Interrupting PPI therapy abruptly may lead to exaggerated rebound gastric acid secretion and rapid development of peptic complications. In patients with high clinical suspicion of ZES, slow weaning off PPI is appropriate to avoid complications. In addition, patients should undergo fasting gastric pH testing.

C. If gastric pH levels are >2, then the condition is not consistent with ZES. The cause of elevated gastrin level could be atrophic gastritis, chronic kidney disease, or due to acid suppression.

D. If gastric pH levels are ≤2 and FSG is elevated ≥10-fold, this is consistent with ZES.

E. If gastric pH levels are ≤2 and FSG is elevated <10-fold, a secretin stimulation test should be performed. The secretin test relies on the finding that IV secretin leads to the secretion of exaggerated amounts of gastrin from gastrinomas, a finding that is likely caused by the presence of specific receptors for secretin on the tumor cells. A positive secretin stimulation test has a high sensitivity (94%) and almost 100% specificity for ZES. An increase in gastrin by at least 120 pg/mL within 5–10 minutes of injecting 2 U/kg of secretin is considered a positive test, and ZES is confirmed.

F. If secretin stimulation test is negative, other causes of elevated serum gastrin and low gastric pH should be considered (gastric outlet obstruction, renal failure, antral G cell hyperplasia, or retained gastric antrum syndrome)

BIBLIOGRAPHY

1. Sleisenger and Fordtran's Gastrointestinal and Liver Disease. 11th Edition. Elsevier, 2020. Chapter 34: Neuroendocrine tumors.
2. Cho MS, Kasi A. Zollinger-Ellison Syndrome. In: StatPearls. Treasure Island (FL): StatPearls Publishing. November;21:202.
3. Dacha S, Razvi M, Massaad J, Cai Q, Wehbi M. Hypergastrinemia Gastroenterol Rep (Oxf). 2015;3(3):201-208. https://doi.org/10.1093/gastro/gov004.

ALGORITHM 27.1 Flowchart for the workup of suspected Zollinger-Ellison syndrome (ZES). *GERD*, Gastroesophageal reflux disease.

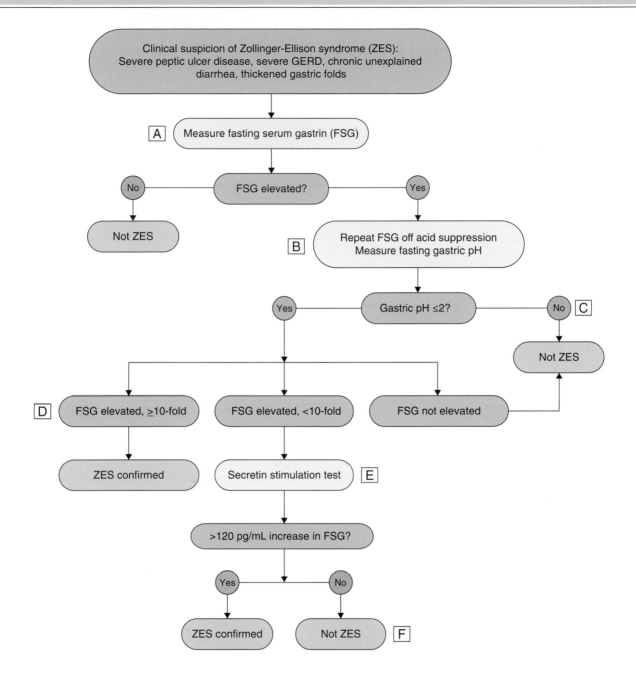

28 Gastric Intestinal Metaplasia

Emad Qayed

Gastric intestinal metaplasia (GIM) is a precursor lesion of gastric cancer, in which the normal gastric epithelium is replaced with intestinal-type epithelium. GIM is strongly associated with *Helicobacter pylori* gastritis and is identified histologically as incomplete (partial colonic type) and complete (small intestinal type) metaplasia. In complete GIM, the cell morphology is similar to the small intestine, with clear brush border with goblet cells. This type does not increase the risk for gastric adenocarcinoma. In incomplete GIM, there is absence of brush borders and difficult-to-identify enterocytes. Incomplete GIM is associated with a 20-fold increased risk of gastric adenocarcinoma. The importance of this lesion stems from its association with the risk of progression to gastric adenocarcinoma. The Correa pathway describes the pathologic steps in the progression to gastric adenocarcinoma (Normal gastric mucosa → superficial gastritis due to *H. pylori* → Atrophic gastritis → GIM of complete type → GIM of incomplete type → Dysplasia → Adenocarcinoma). Surveillance with esophagogastroduodenoscopy (EGD) is reasonable in patients with GIM at higher risk of developing gastric cancer, such as those with incomplete type GIM, extensive GIM that involves the gastric body, family history of gastric cancer, and persistent *H. pylori* infection. Surveillance should also be considered in patients who have an overall higher risk of gastric cancer, such as racial/ethnic minorities and immigrants from high-incidence regions.

A. GIM is often diagnosed during routine EGD performed for various indications in which a gastric biopsy is obtained. During the index exam, random biopsies are usually obtained from the antrum and body and placed in one jar; therefore, if the histology shows GIM, it would be unclear if the GIM is extensive (involving the body and antrum) or limited (involving the antrum alone).

B. If the index EGD is inadequate, then a repeat EGD should be performed. In patients with GIM, a high-quality endoscopy with full visualization of the mucosa is essential to examine for precancerous lesions and early gastric cancer. Some physicians would repeat the endoscopy in all patients with GIM to exclude prevalent gastric precursor lesions or gastric cancer. The repeat endoscopy would focus more on meticulous mucosal inspection, photodocumentation of all parts of the stomach (antrum; lower, mid, and upper gastric body; incisura; fundus; and cardia), and utilization of image-enhanced endoscopy to examine suspicious areas. Any abnormal mucosa should be clearly and accurately described and biopsied separately. Therefore, repeat EGD within 1 year should be considered in all patients with GIM. To document the extent of GIM, "gastric mapping" should be performed, and biopsies should be obtained from the gastric antrum and body and placed in separate jars.

C. *H. pylori* infection should be treated adequately and eradication confirmed. Further consideration of surveillance EGD depends on the presence of risk factors for progression to gastric cancer.

D. Patients with any risk factor should be offered EGD in 3 years if they are reasonable candidates for endoscopy with good life expectancy.

E. Patients without any risk factor do not need surveillance EGD.

F. Patients without known risk factors in whom the extent of GIM is unknown should undergo repeat EGD for gastric mapping if they are otherwise in good health and with reasonable life expectancy.

G. Patients with extensive GIM should be offered surveillance, while those with limited GIM to the antrum do not need surveillance.

BIBLIOGRAPHY

1. Gupta S, Li D, El Serag HB, et al. AGA clinical practice guidelines on management of gastric intestinal metaplasia. *Gastroenterology*. 2020;158(3):693-702. https://doi.org/10.1053/j.gastro.2019.12.003.
2. Banks M, Graham D, Jansen M, et al. British Society of Gastroenterology guidelines on the diagnosis and management of patients at risk of gastric adenocarcinoma. *Gut*. 2019;68(9):1545-1575. https://doi.org/10.1136/gutjnl-2018-318126.
3. Sleisenger, Fordtran's Gastrointestinal, Liver Disease, 11th Edition. Elsevier, 2021. Chapter 54: Adenocarcinoma of the Stomach and Other Gastric Tumors.

ALGORITHM 28.1 Flowchart for the management of gastric intestinal metaplasia. *EGD*, Esophagogastroduodenoscopy; *GIM*, gastric intestinal metaplasia; *H. pylori*, Helicobacter pylori.

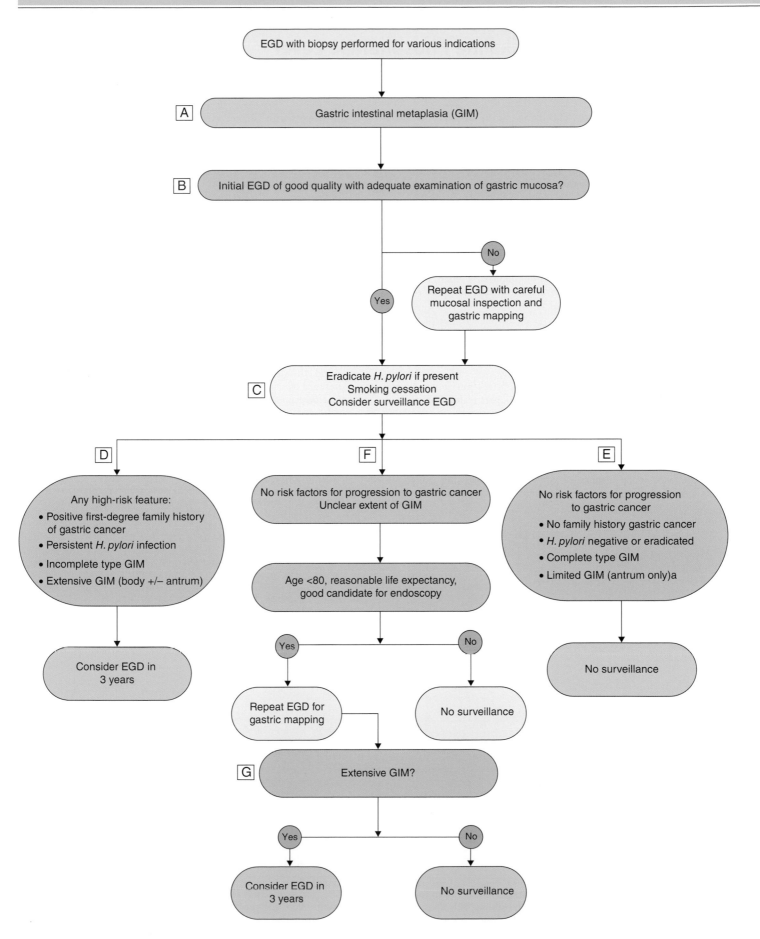

EGD with biopsy performed for various indications

A — Gastric intestinal metaplasia (GIM)

B — Initial EGD of good quality with adequate examination of gastric mucosa?

No → Repeat EGD with careful mucosal inspection and gastric mapping

Yes

C — Eradicate *H. pylori* if present
Smoking cessation
Consider surveillance EGD

D — Any high-risk feature:
- Positive first-degree family history of gastric cancer
- Persistent *H. pylori* infection
- Incomplete type GIM
- Extensive GIM (body +/– antrum)

Consider EGD in 3 years

F — No risk factors for progression to gastric cancer
Unclear extent of GIM

Age <80, reasonable life expectancy, good candidate for endoscopy

Yes → Repeat EGD for gastric mapping

No → No surveillance

G — Extensive GIM?

Yes → Consider EGD in 3 years

No → No surveillance

E — No risk factors for progression to gastric cancer
- No family history gastric cancer
- *H. pylori* negative or eradicated
- Complete type GIM
- Limited GIM (antrum only)a

No surveillance

29 Elevated Alkaline Phosphatase Level

Nikrad Shahnavaz

Hepatic alkaline phosphatase (ALP) is one of the various ALP isoenzymes in humans. It is found on the canalicular membrane of hepatocytes, and its exact function remains unknown. Elevated ALP level is sensitive for detection of intrahepatic or extrahepatic bile duct obstruction, and ALP has a serum half-life of 7 days. The elevated serum ALP level is caused by increased production during biliary obstruction rather than leakage from bile duct cells or failure to clear circulating ALP.

A. Nonhepatic ALP isoenzymes originate from bone, intestine, kidney, and placenta. Elevations are seen in Paget disease of the bone, osteoblastic bone metastases, small intestinal obstruction, pregnancy, or normal postprandial status. Normal levels of ALP are higher during children's growth years and also in middle-aged women, peaking at the age of 65 years. When ALP level is elevated, it should be repeated while fasting (if not done before).

B. A hepatic origin of an elevated ALP level is confirmed by simultaneous elevation of either serum gamma-glutamyltranspeptidase (GGTP) or 5′-nucleotidase (5NT).

C. If abdominal ultrasound is concerning for obstruction from malignancy or stone, endoscopic retrograde cholangiopancreatography (ERCP) is preferred as a diagnostic and potentially therapeutic modality. In chronic cholestatic conditions without any obvious etiology of obstruction identified during ultrasound, MRCP is the preferred choice.

D. In patients newly diagnosed with primary sclerosing cholangitis, colonoscopy is performed to rule out inflammatory bowel disease or colon cancer.

E. In patients with isolated elevation of ALP and normal abdominal ultrasound, further workup is needed to evaluate for primary biliary cholangitis, granulomatous disease like sarcoidosis and viral hepatitis. The angiotensin-converting enzyme (ACE) test is used to help in the diagnosis of sarcoidosis.

F. The presence of antimitochondrial antibody (AMA) and normal ultrasound is strongly suggestive of primary biliary cholangitis. Liver biopsy is performed to confirm the diagnosis and assess for the presence of cirrhosis.

G. If ALP levels remain elevated for 6 months or longer, and the workup is nondiagnostic, liver biopsy is recommended to rule out granulomatous infections, sarcoidosis, malignancy, or idiopathic bile ductopenia. If liver biopsy is non-diagnostic, the patient needs to be monitored closely with liver function tests and abdominal ultrasound performed every 3–6 months.

H. If gallstone is found during the right upper quadrant (RUQ) ultrasound, the decision for cholecystectomy should be based on the presence of symptoms (biliary pain) and findings suggestive of bile duct obstruction or complications. In asymptomatic patients with gallstone, expectant management is usually recommended.

BIBLIOGRAPHY

1. Pratt DS Liver chemistry and function tests. Sleisenger and Fordtran's Gastrointestinal and Liver Disease, 11th edition. Elsevier; 2020.
2. Martin P, Friedman LS. Assessment of liver function and diagnostic studies. Handbook of Liver Disease. 4th edition 1. Elsevier; 2017.

ALGORITHM 29.1 Evaluation of an isolated elevation of the serum alkaline phosphatase level. *5′NT*, 5′ Nucleotidase; *ACE*, angiotensin-converting enzyme; *ALP*, alkaline phosphatase; *AMA*, antimitochondrial antibody; *CT*, computed tomography; *ERCP*, endoscopic retrograde cholangiopancreatography; *GGTP*, gamma-glutamyl transpeptidase; *MRCP*, magnetic resonance cholangiopancreatography; *MRI*, magnetic resonance imaging; *RUQ*, right upper quadrant.

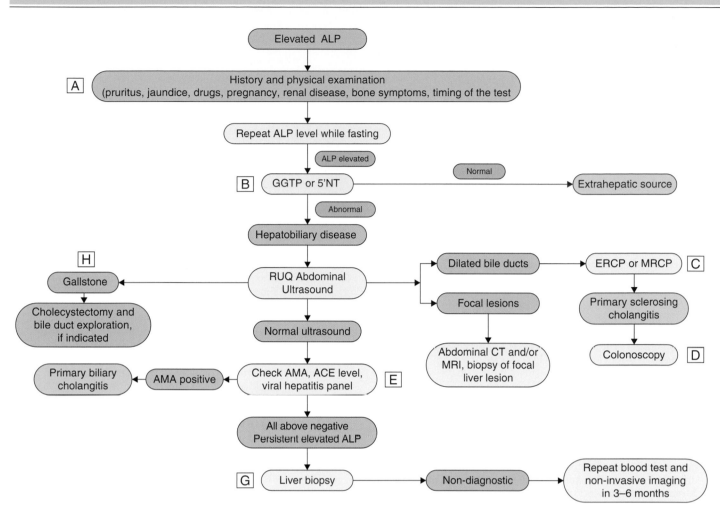

30 Elevated Transaminases

Nikrad Shahnavaz

The serum aminotransferases (alanine transaminase [ALT] and aspartate transaminase [AST]) are the most sensitive markers of acute hepatocellular injury. Although ALT is a more specific indicator of liver injury than AST, they both can be found, in order of decreasing concentration, in liver, cardiac muscle, skeletal muscle, kidney, brain, pancreas, lung, leukocytes, and erythrocytes. Moreover, the magnitude of aminotransferases' elevation in serum does not correlate with the extent of liver injury.

A. Mild elevation (≤5-fold) of ALT and AST is nonspecific and is usually identified during routine screening of asymptomatic patients. In these cases, the first step is to repeat the test to confirm persistence of the elevated values. Marked elevations of aminotransferase levels (>1000 U/L) have a more specific differential diagnosis, which includes viral or ischemic hepatitis, toxin- or drug-induced liver injury, and less commonly, autoimmune hepatitis, acute Budd-Chiari syndrome, acute cholestasis, or acute liver failure caused by Wilson disease. The ratio of AST to ALT in serum is helpful in the diagnoses of alcohol-associated liver disease. If the AST level is less than 300 U/L, a ratio of AST to ALT of more than 2 is suggestive of alcohol-associated liver disease. The higher AST levels compared to ALT have been attributed to reduced ALT activity due to hepatic B6 depletion and mitochondrial damage from alcohol intake leading to increased release of mitochondrial AST in serum.

B. Once the elevated values of AST and ALT are confirmed, a focused history should be obtained to document the patient's medications, drinking habits, and any substance abuse. Medications that frequently cause liver injury include antibiotics, statins, antiepileptics, nonsteroidal antiinflammatory drugs (NSAIDs), and antituberculosis medications. Also, over-the-counter medications including herbal supplements are common unrecognized causes of liver injury.

C. The association between an agent use and liver enzyme elevations could be established by discontinuing the toxin/medication and witnessing the normalization of the liver enzymes in 3–4 months. Rechallenge with the suspect medication is rarely necessary and is not advised.

D. In patients with myalgia, muscle weakness, or exercise intolerance, creatine kinase and aldolase levels should be checked to exclude muscular sources of elevated AST and ALT.

E. The next step after excluding medications and toxins as the cause of transaminitis is to evaluate the patient for common causes of liver injury which include nonalcoholic fatty liver disease (most common cause in the United States), viral hepatitis, autoimmune hepatitis, hereditary hemochromatosis, and Wilson disease (in patients younger than 40 years old).

F. The diagnosis of autoimmune hepatitis is suspected with positive anti–smooth muscle antibody (ASMA), antinuclear antibodies (ANAs), and increased immunoglobulin G (IgG) levels in the serum, but it needs to be confirmed with liver biopsy in most cases.

G. When history and studies for the more common causes of elevated AST and ALT are nondiagnostic, the less common causes of liver disease, such as α_1-antitrypsin deficiency, and extrahepatic causes, such as celiac disease, thyroid disease, and adrenal insufficiency, should be ruled out in patients with persistently elevated liver enzyme levels.

H. In patients with prolonged elevation of AST and ALT (more than twice the upper limit of normal) and nondiagnostic studies as earlier, liver biopsy should be considered. Liver biopsy may aid in the diagnosis and management of patients with asymptomatic elevation of liver enzymes and negative serological markers. Examples of etiologies uncovered by liver biopsy include nonalcoholic steatohepatitis, fatty liver disease, cryptogenic hepatitis, drug-induced liver injury, alcoholic liver disease, and autoimmune hepatitis.

BIBLIOGRAPHY

1. Pratt DS Liver chemistry and function tests. Sleisenger and Fordtran's Gastrointestinal and Liver Disease. Elsevier; 2020. 11th ed.
2. Martin P, Friedman LS Assessment of liver function and diagnostic studies. Handbook of Liver Disease. Elsevier; 2017. 4th ed.
3. Habib S, Shaikh OS Approach to jaundice and abnormal liver function test results. Zakim and Boyer's Hepatology. Elsevier; 2016. 7th ed.
4. Skelly MM, James PD, Ryder SD Findings on liver biopsy to investigate abnormal liver function tests in the absence of diagnostic serology. J Hepatol. 2001;35(2):195-199. https://doi.org/10.1016/s0168-8278(01)00094-0.

ALGORITHM 30.1 Evaluation of elevated transaminases. α_1-*AT*, α_1-Antitrypsin; *ANA*, antinuclear antibody; *Anti-HBc*, antibody to hepatitis B core antigen; *Anti-HBe*, antibody to hepatitis B e antigen; *Anti-HBs*, antibody to hepatitis B surface antigen; *Anti-HCV*, antibody to HCV; *HBeAg*, hepatitis B e antigen; *HBsAg*, hepatitis B surface antigen; *HBV*, hepatitis B virus; *HCV*, hepatitis C virus; *HFE*, hemochromatosis; *IgG*, immunoglobulin G; *OTC*, over the counter; *RUQ US*, right upper quadrant ultrasound; *SMA*, smooth muscle antibodies; *SPEP*, serum protein electrophoresis; *TIBC*, total iron binding capacity; *TFTs*, thyroid function tests; *TTG*, tissue transglutaminase; *ULN*, upper limit of normal.

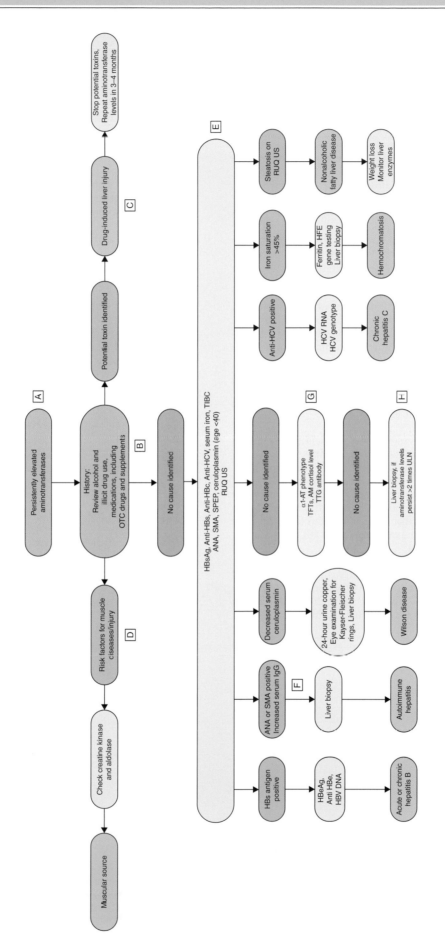

Persistently elevated aminotransferases **A**

History: Review alcohol and illicit drug use, medications, including OTC drugs and supplements **B**

Potential toxin identified

Drug-induced liver injury **C**

Stop potential toxins, Repeat aminotransferase levels in 3–4 months

No cause identified

HBsAg, Anti-HBs, Anti-HBc, Anti-HCV, serum iron, TIBC ANA, SMA, SPEP, ceruloplasmin (age <40) RUQ US **E**

Risk factors for muscle diseases/injury **D**

Check creatine kinase and aldolase

Muscular source

HBs antigen positive → HBeAg, Anti HBe, HBV DNA → Acute or chronic hepatitis B

ANA or SMA positive Increased serum IgG → Liver biopsy **F** → Autoimmune hepatitis

Decreased serum ceruloplasmin → 24-hour urine copper, Eye examination for Kayser-Fleischer rings, Liver biopsy → Wilson disease

Anti-HCV positive → HCV RNA HCV genotype → Chronic hepatitis C

Iron saturation >45% → Ferritin, HFE gene testing Liver biopsy → Hemochromatosis

Steatosis on RUQ US → Nonalcoholic fatty liver disease → Weight loss Monitor liver enzymes

No cause identified

α1-AT phenotype TFTs, AM cortisol level TTG antibody **G**

No cause identified

Liver biopsy, if aminotransferase levels persist >2 times ULN **F**

31 Drug-Induced Liver Injury (DILI)

Nikrad Shahnavaz

Drug-induced liver injury (DILI) is a common condition encountered by gastroenterologists and hepatologists in their practice, and yet, it could be a diagnostic challenge due to its diverse presentations, long list of culprit medications/supplements, and the absence of objective diagnostic tests. Intrinsic DILI is dose dependent in a predictable pattern (acetaminophen toxicity), while idiosyncratic DILI is only seen in susceptible individuals, has more diverse manifestation, and is less associated with the dosage of the culprit agent.

A. The most important aspects of the evaluation and diagnosis of patients with possible DILI are history of drug exposure in relation to the onset and the course of liver enzyme abnormality. Antibiotics and antiepileptics, followed by analgesics (nonsteroidal antiinflammatory drugs [NSAIDs]), immune modulators and checkpoint inhibitors, androgen-containing steroids, amiodarone, methotrexate, and allopurinol, are the most common culprit medications to cause DILI. In addition, a thorough history of herbal and dietary supplements (HDSs) and over-the-counter drug consumption needs to be collected. The clinical presentation of DILI ranges from asymptomatic elevation in the liver enzymes to systemic symptoms including nausea, vomiting, abdominal pain, jaundice, pruritus, malaise, and encephalopathy. Physical examination is mostly focused on finding any evidence of acute or chronic liver failure.

B. R-ratio can be calculated at presentation to differentiate the pattern of liver injury to hepatocellular, cholestatic, or mixed patterns. It is calculated as serum alanine aminotransferase (ALT)/ALT upper limit of normal (ULN) divided by serum alkaline phosphatase (ALP)/ALP ULN. The differential diagnosis and further workup will be guided by the pattern of the liver injury. This is particularly valuable in excluding other conditions that could mimic DILI. On the other hand, the same medication can potentially cause DILI with varying patterns in different individuals.

C. In patients with hepatocellular or mixed patterns, the next step would be to check for anti-hepatitis A virus (HAV) antibody, anti-hepatitis B surface (HBs) antigen, anti-HBs antibody, anti-hepatitis B core (HBc) antibody, anti-hepatitis C virus (HCV) antibody, antinuclear anibody (ANA), anti-smooth muscle antibody (ASMA), anti-liver-kidney microsomal-1 antibody (Ani-LKM-1), gamma globulin levels, as well as right upper quadrant ultrasound with doppler to rule out common causes of hepatotoxicity such as viral, autoimmune hepatitis, portal vein thrombosis, or Budd-Chiari syndrome. Of note, patients with hypersensitivity reactions to medications may present with positive ANA or peripheral eosinophilia within the first 72 hours after exposure to the culprit drug.

D. If the workup for common causes of hepatotoxicity is nondiagnostic, further testings for less common infectious causes or Wilson disease should be considered in special cases with known risk factors or supporting clinical manifestations.

E. Liver biopsy can supplement the workup of DILI by excluding or confirming other possible causes of liver injury. However, liver biopsy is not universally required for the diagnosis of DILI. Persistence of liver test abnormality and high suspicion for autoimmune hepatitis are the main reasons to consider liver biopsy during the workup of DILI. Furthermore, liver biopsy can be considered in rare occasions where continued use or rechallenge of a particular medicine is clinically necessary.

F. Final diagnosis of DILI is made only after non-DILI etiologies are reasonably ruled out and after complete assessment of available clinical data and literature review using LiverTox and PubMed database. Expert consultation may be needed in challenging situations.

BIBLIOGRAPHY

1. Chalasani NP, Maddur H, Russo MW, Wong RJ, Rajender Reddy K. Practice Parameters Committee of the American College of Gastroenterology. ACG clinical guideline: diagnosis and management of idiosyncratic drug-induced liver injury. *Am J Gastroenterol.* 2021;116(5):878-898.
2. Sandhu N, Navarro V. Drug-induced liver injury in GI practice. *Hepatol Commun.* 2020;4(5):631-645.
3. Sleisenger and Fordtran's Gastrointestinal and Liver Disease, 11th Edition, 2020. Chapter 88, Liver disease caused by drugs.

ALGORITHM 31.1 Evaluation of drug induced liver injury. *AIH,* Autoimmune hepatitis; *ALP,* alkaline phosphatase; *ALT,* alanine aminotransferase; *CMV,* Cytomegalovirus; *DILI,* drug-induced liver injury; *EBV,* Epstein–Barr virus; *ERCP,* endoscopic retrograde cholangiopancreatography; *HCV,* hepatitis C virus; *HEV,* hepatitis E virus; *HSV,* herpes simplex virus; *MRCP,* magnetic resonance cholangiopancreatography; *ULN,* upper limit of normal.

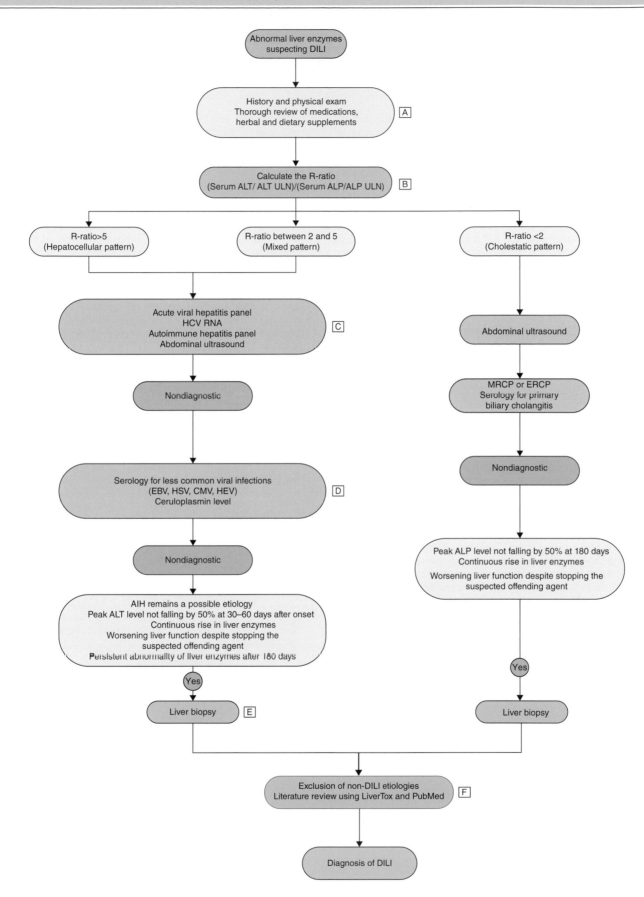

Management of Hepatitis B

Anand S. Shah

Chronic hepatitis B virus (HBV) infection has been on the decline due to vaccination and use of antiviral therapy–nucleoside analog treatment (NAT). Chronic HBV infection can cause progressive liver disease through active viral replication and necroinflammation of the liver, ultimately resulting in advanced fibrosis, cirrhosis, and hepatocellular carcinoma (HCC). Management of HBV infection first starts with testing for hepatitis B surface antigen (HBsAg) in those with abnormalities in liver chemistries, perinatally, and high-risk populations. Currently, the Centers for Disease Control and Prevention (CDC) recommends screening for hepatitis B in all adults at least once during their lifetime. Further management of HBV depends on the presence of cirrhosis, HBV DNA level, and alanine transaminase (ALT) level. Patients who qualify for treatment are usually given NAT; however, peginterferon alfa can be used in patients without cirrhosis or with well-compensated cirrhosis.

A. The initial step in the management of HBV is to perform a comprehensive history and assess for high-risk behaviors, transmissibility, and family history of liver disease or liver cancer. Physical examination can aid in diagnosing advanced liver disease. Laboratory examination of liver chemistries, hepatitis B core immunoglobulin G (IgG) antibody, hepatitis B E antigen (HBeAg), hepatitis B E antibody (anti-HBe), and HBV DNA level should be carried out. The degree of liver fibrosis should be assessed by noninvasive testing such as elastography and/or ultrasound and, in certain cases, liver biopsy. Patients with human immunodeficiency virus (HIV) coinfection should receive treatment for both HIV and HBV and are usually referred to infectious disease specialists for treatment.

B. In patients with stage 3 fibrosis or compensated cirrhosis (stage 4 fibrosis), long-term NAT with entecavir, tenofovir alafenamide (TAF), or tenofovir disoproxil fumarate (TDF) is recommended. Patients who develop HBsAg loss for 6–12 months or HBsAg seroconversion may stop therapy, but they require long-term surveillance for HCC. If there is decompensated cirrhosis, long-term NAT with entecavir or TDF should be started along with liver transplant evaluation. TAF is not recommended in decompensated cirrhosis.

C. If there is no evidence of advanced fibrosis or cirrhosis, then management should be based on HBV DNA level and ALT level. If HBV DNA is <2000 IU/mL and ALT is normal, then it is recommended to assess ALT and HBV DNA every 6–12 months, and NAT is not indicated. If ALT becomes elevated, consider further workup for concurrent causes of liver disease such as hepatitis C, hepatitis D, autoimmune hepatitis, alcohol liver disease, nonalcoholic fatty liver disease, hemochromatosis, Wilson disease, and A1 antitrypsin disease.

D. *HBV chronic hepatitis* is defined as having HBV DNA levels >2000 IU/mL and an elevated ALT—defined as >35 IU/mL in men and >25 IU/mL in women without cirrhosis or advanced fibrosis. HBV *chronic infection*, previously called "immune tolerant stage", is defined as having HBV DNA >2000 IU/mL and a normal ALT level.

E. Management of HBV chronic infection further depends on HBeAg status. If HBeAg is positive, then entecavir or TAF should be considered in patients with high-risk factors for developing HCC, young age, high-risk lifestyle for transmission, high risk of reactivation, or a desire to undergo treatment.

F. If HBeAg is negative in HBV chronic infection, then ALT should be monitored every 3–6 months along with intermittent fibrosis assessment. If ALT becomes elevated or fibrosis is present, then consider initiation of NAT.

G. In HBV chronic hepatitis, NAT with entecavir, TDF, or TAF should be initiated with the goal of long-term HBV DNA suppression and normalization of ALT. In patients without HBsAg seroconversion, treatment should be continued long term.

BIBLIOGRAPHY

1. Terrault NA, Lok ASF, McMahon BJ, et al. Update on prevention, diagnosis, and treatment of chronic hepatitis B: AASLD 2018 hepatitis B guidance. *Hepatology.* 2018;67(4):1560-1599. https://doi.org/10.1002/hep.29800.
2. European Association for the Study of the Liver. EASL 2017 Clinical Practice Guidelines on the management of hepatitis B virus infection. *J Hepatol.* 2017;67(2):370-398. https://doi.org/10.1016/j.jhep.2017.03.021.
3. Martin P, Nguyen MH, Dieterich DT, et al. Treatment algorithm for managing chronic hepatitis B virus infection in the United States: 2021 update. *Clin Gastroenterol Hepatol.* 2022;20(8):1766-1775. https://doi.org/10.1016/j.cgh.2021.07.036.

ALGORITHM 32.1 Flowchart for the workup and management of patients with chronic hepatitis B virus infection (HBV). *ALT,* Alanine transaminase; *anti-HBe,* hepatitis B E antibody; *HBeAg,* hepatitis B E antigen; *HBsAg,* hepatitis B surface antigen; *HCC,* hepatocellular carcinoma; *NAT,* nucleoside analog treatment; *TAF,* tenofovir alafenamide; *TDF,* tenofovir disoproxil fumarate.

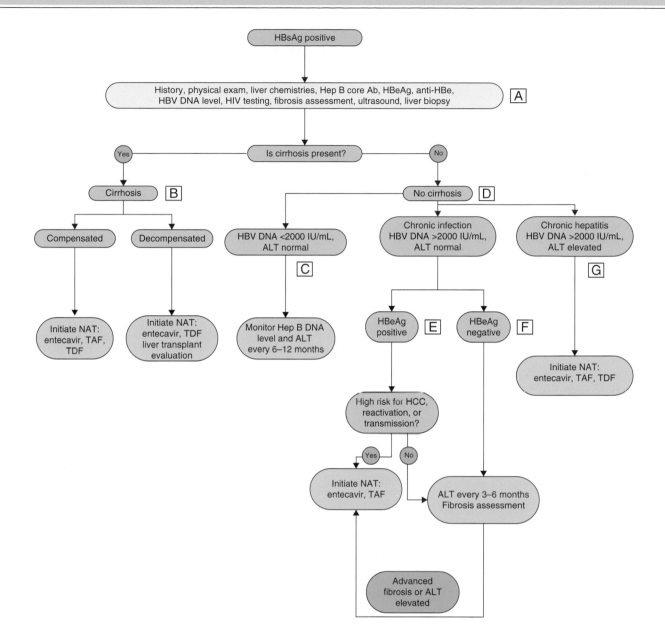

33 | Treatment of Hepatitis B during Pregnancy

Anand S. Shah

Screening for hepatitis B virus (HBV) infection should be performed in the first trimester of pregnancy. Patients found to be hepatitis B surface antigen (HBsAg) positive during pregnancy require additional workup and evaluation. The goal is to minimize mother-to-child transmission.

A. The initial step is the same as management of HBV (see Chapter 32). Perform a comprehensive history and assess for high-risk behaviors, transmissibility, and family history of liver disease or liver cancer. Physical examination can aid in diagnosing advanced liver disease. Laboratory examination of liver chemistries, hepatitis B core IgG antibody, hepatitis B core IgM antibody, hepatitis B E antigen (HBeAg), hepatitis B E antibody (anti-HBe), and HBV DNA level should be obtained.

B. If there is an indication for treatment outside of pregnancy, such as evidence of elevation of alanine transaminase (ALT) and HBV DNA, greater than mild liver inflammation, greater than mild fibrosis, or cirrhosis, then nucleoside analog treatment (NAT) should be initiated or continued to manage maternal liver disease and prevent obstetric complications. NAT options considered safe in pregnancy include tenofovir disoproxil fumarate, telbivudine, and lamivudine.

C. If the HBV DNA reaches greater than 200,000 IU/mL by 28 to 32 weeks' gestation, then NAT should be initiated. High-risk situations for maternal-to-child transmission include previous infant with immunoprophylaxis failure, premature rupture of membranes, preterm labor, or invasive testing such as amniocentesis. NAT is considered in these situations.

D. If there is an indication for the HBsAg-positive person to continue HBV treatment (as described in Chapter 32) after childbirth, then

NAT is continued. Adverse events for continuing NAT have not been observed in breastfeeding. If there is no indication to continue NAT, it can be safely discontinued after delivery.

E. If the HBV DNA is <200,000 IU/mL by 28 to 32 weeks' gestation and without a high-risk situation for maternal-child transmission, then HBV DNA level and ALT can be monitored until birth.

F. All infants born to patients with HBsAg positivity should receive hepatitis B immune globulin (HBIG) and the first dose of HBV vaccine within 12 hours of birth. Cesarean section is not routinely recommended to reduce perinatal HBV transmission. Infants could be breastfed after receiving HBIG and HBV vaccine at birth.

BIBLIOGRAPHY

1. Terrault NA, Lok ASF, McMahon BJ, et al. Update on prevention, diagnosis, and treatment of chronic hepatitis B: AASLD 2018 hepatitis B guidance. *Hepatology*. 2018;67(4):1560-1599. https://doi.org/10.1002/hep.29800.
2. European Association for the Study of the Liver. EASL 2017 Clinical Practice Guidelines on the management of hepatitis B virus infection. *J Hepatol*. 2017;67(2):370-398. https://doi.org/10.1016/j.jhep.2017.03.021.
3. Brown Jr RS, McMahon BJ, Lok AS, et al. Antiviral therapy in chronic hepatitis B viral infection during pregnancy: A systematic review and meta-analysis. *Hepatology*. 2016;63(1):319-333. https://doi.org/10.1002/hep.28302.
4. Zou H, Chen Y, Duan Z, Zhang H, Pan C. Virologic factors associated with failure to passive-active immunoprophylaxis in infants born to HBsAg-positive mothers. *J Viral Hepat*. 2012;19(2):e18-e25. https://doi.org/10.1111/j.1365-2893.2011.01492.x.

ALGORITHM 33.1 Flowchart for the treatment of HBV in pregnancy. ALT, Alanine transaminase; *HBIG*, hepatitis B immune globulin; *HBV*, hepatitis B virus; *NAT*, nucleoside analog treatment.

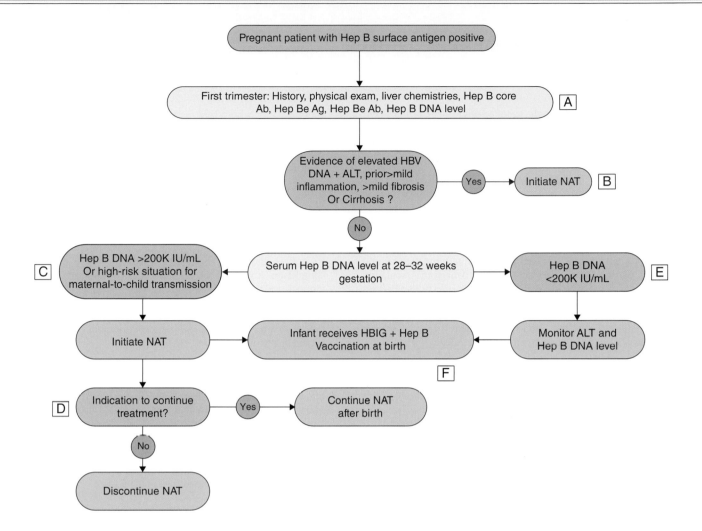

34 Management of Hepatitis C

Emad Qayed

Hepatitis C virus (HCV) is a single-stranded RNA virus of the Flaviviridae family of viruses. The majority of patients infected with HCV will develop chronic infection, and many will progress to cirrhosis and develop hepatocellular carcinoma. The worldwide prevalence of HCV infection is estimated to be 0.7%, with approximately 57 million people infected chronically. Given the global burden of disease, screening and treatment for HCV is essential to prevent complications of chronic infection. The United States Preventive Services Task Force (USPSTF) recommends screening for HCV in all adults aged 18–79 years. Treatment of HCV infection has been revolutionized by the development of highly efficacious direct-acting antiviral drugs. These drugs enabled the creation of highly potent and well-tolerated interferon-free all-oral treatment regimens with cure rates of >95%. The American Association for the Study of Liver Diseases (AASLD) and the Infectious Diseases Society of America (IDSA) have developed simplified treatment regimens that can be administered safely by any provider knowledgeable about HCV. Patients with HCV who have characteristics that require other regimens should be referred to an HCV specialist.

A. Patients with chronic HCV infection should have a clinical evaluation with a complete history, physical exam, and basic workup to assess for cirrhosis and other clinical comorbidities. The presence of cirrhosis can be diagnosed based on clinical, imaging, and laboratory findings (e.g., ascites, encephalopathy, bleeding, liver nodularity on ultrasound or cross-sectional imaging, splenomegaly, and low platelets). Other tests for cirrhosis include calculating the FIB-4 score (>3.25 indicates cirrhosis), liver stiffness measurements (e.g., transient elastography), and other noninvasive serologic liver fibrosis tests.

B. Based on the initial assessment, patients with any of these listed characteristics are not eligible for this simplified treatment regimen and should be considered for other regimens. Of note, patients with compensated cirrhosis (Child-Turcotte-Pugh class A with total score of ≤6) who have not received prior treatment for HCV may qualify for another simplified treatment regimen published by the IDSA and AASLD (HCVGuidelines.org). This regimen consists of glecaprevir (300 mg) with pibrentasvir (120 mg) taken with food for 8 weeks for Genotypes 1–6. An alternative regimen for Genotype 1, 2, 4, 5, or 6 is sofosbuvir (400 mg)/velpatasvir (100 mg) for a duration of 12 weeks. In patients with compensated cirrhosis and HCV genotype 3 for whom treatment with sofosbuvir/velpatasvir is considered, it is necessary to test for baseline NS5A resistance-associated substitution (RAS). If RAS Y93H is absent, then patients can receive sofosbuvir/velpatasvir regimen. If Y93H is present, other treatment regimens should be considered.

C. Patients without any of these listed characteristics are eligible for treatment with these simplified regimens, which can be used in all HCV genotypes. The patient's medication history should be carefully recorded to assess for any potential drug-drug interaction assessment.

D. HCV RNA should be checked at 12 weeks or later after treatment completion. If HCV RNA is undetectable, this indicates sustained virologic response (virologic cure).

E. If liver transaminase levels have normalized, no specific liver-related follow-up is required. Otherwise, then workup for other liver disease should be conducted.

F. If sustained virologic response is not achieved, the patient should be referred to a liver specialist for consideration of retreatment with other regimens. Management options include treatment with the same or a different baseline regimen, combined with additional antivirals (e.g., voxilaprevir, ribavirin, and sofosbuvir) for 12–16 weeks.

BIBLIOGRAPHY

1. HCV Guidance: Recommendations for Testing, Managing, and Treating Hepatitis C. https://www.hcvguidelines.org/. Accessed 7/17/2023.
2. Ghany MG, Morgan TR, AASLD-IDSA Hepatitis C Guidance Panel. Hepatitis C guidance 2019 update: American Association for the Study of Liver Diseases–Infectious Diseases Society of America recommendations for testing, managing, and treating hepatitis C virus infection. *Hepatology.* 2020;71(2):686-721. https://doi.org/10.1002/hep.31060.
3. Polaris Observatory HCV Collaborators. Global change in hepatitis C virus prevalence and cascade of care between 2015 and 2020: a modelling study. *Lancet Gastroenterol Hepatol.* 2022;7(5):396-415. https://doi.org/10.1016/S2468-1253(21)00472-6.
4. Preventive Services Task Force US, Owens DK, Davidson KW Screening for hepatitis C virus infection in adolescents and adults: US Preventive Services Task Force recommendation statement. *JAMA.* 2020;323(10):970-975.
5. Sleisenger and Fordtran's Gastrointestinal and Liver Disease, Eleventh Edition, Elsevier, 2021. Chapter 80, Hepatitis C.

ALGORITHM 34.1 Flowchart for the workup and management of treatment-naïve patients with chronic hepatitis C without cirrhosis. *CBC,* Complete blood count; *HBsAg,* hepatitis B surface antigen; *HCV,* hepatitis C virus; *HIV,* human immunodeficiency virus.

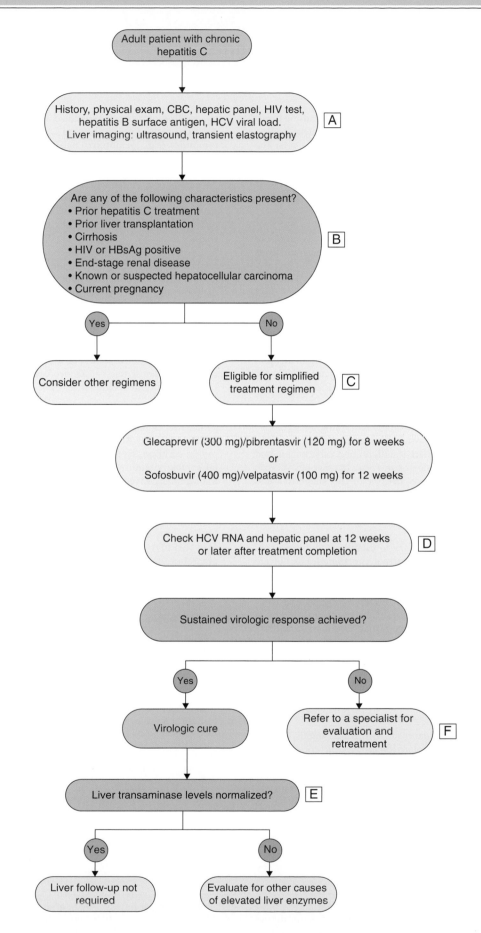

Adult patient with chronic hepatitis C

History, physical exam, CBC, hepatic panel, HIV test, hepatitis B surface antigen, HCV viral load. Liver imaging: ultrasound, transient elastography | A

Are any of the following characteristics present?
• Prior hepatitis C treatment
• Prior liver transplantation
• Cirrhosis
• HIV or HBsAg positive
• End-stage renal disease
• Known or suspected hepatocellular carcinoma
• Current pregnancy | B

Yes

No

Consider other regimens

Eligible for simplified treatment regimen | C

Glecaprevir (300 mg)/pibrentasvir (120 mg) for 8 weeks
or
Sofosbuvir (400 mg)/velpatasvir (100 mg) for 12 weeks

Check HCV RNA and hepatic panel at 12 weeks or later after treatment completion | D

Sustained virologic response achieved?

Yes

No

Virologic cure

Refer to a specialist for evaluation and retreatment | F

Liver transaminase levels normalized? | E

Yes

No

Liver follow-up not required

Evaluate for other causes of elevated liver enzymes

35 Primary Sclerosing Cholangitis

Nikrad Shahnavaz

Sclerosing cholangitis refers to a broad range of disorders causing fibrosis of the bile ducts, usually of medium-sized and large ducts, leading to segmental strictures with proximal dilatation of the bile ducts. The diagnosis of primary sclerosing cholangitis (PSC) is confirmed when the characteristic findings of beading and stricture formation of the bile ducts cannot be attributed to another inflammatory, infectious, or malignant underlying cause, thus differentiating PSC from secondary sclerosing cholangitis.

A. Cholestatic profile of liver tests with predominant elevation of alkaline phosphatase (ALP) and gamma-glutamyl transferase levels along with modestly elevated aspartate transaminase (AST) and alanine transaminase (ALT) are usually seen.

B. In patients with persistent cholestatic liver tests, the next step is right upper quadrant (RUQ) abdominal ultrasound to exclude biliary obstruction caused by stone or malignancy. If checked, antimitochondrial antibody (AMA), which is characteristic of primary biliary cholangitis (PBC), is not found in PSC. However, antineutrophil cytoplasmic antibodies (ANCA) (specifically perinuclear ANCA, or pANCA) are detected in up to 88% of patients with PSC.

C. Magnetic resonance cholangiopancreatography (MRCP) has largely supplanted endoscopic retrograde cholangiopancreatography (ERCP) as the first-line diagnostic test when PSC is suspected; however, ERCP should be considered if there is a high index of suspicion and MRCP findings are not diagnostic or equivocal. In cases of PSC with a dominant stricture, ERCP is indicated for further diagnostic and therapeutic interventions such as brush cytology, intraductal biopsy, cholangioscopy for the diagnosis of cholangiocarcinoma, as well as balloon dilation of strictures and biliary stent placement.

D. Liver biopsy is generally not necessary to establish the diagnosis of PSC, except in patients who have normal cholangiograms but are suspected to have small-duct PSC in the setting of unexplained cholestasis. Small-duct PSC may represent an early stage of classic PSC; however, it is usually associated with better long-term prognosis than classic PSC. A characteristic finding on liver biopsy in PSC is a fibro-obliterative process that can lead to an "onion-skin" appearance with concentric fibrosis surrounding medium-sized bile ducts. This finding is present in <50% of patients. If this process involves the smaller interlobular and septal bile duct branches, these ducts become entirely obliterated by this process (fibro-obliterative cholangitis), a finding that is seen in 5%–10% of biopsy samples but is considered pathognomonic of PSC.

E. Common etiologies for secondary sclerosing cholangitis include infectious disorders (AIDS cholangiopathy, recurrent pyogenic cholangitis), cholangiocarcinoma, diffuse intrahepatic malignancy (lymphoma), sarcoidosis, intraarterial chemotherapy, ischemia resulting from surgical complication, hepatic artery thrombosis, trauma, or vasculitis. Recently, SARS-CoV-2-2019 (COVID-19)

severe illness has been associated with progressive cholestasis and secondary sclerosing cholangitis. Drugs such as immune checkpoint inhibitors (e.g., pembrolizumab) and recreational ketamine have been associated with sclerosing cholangitis.

F. All patients diagnosed with PSC should be tested for elevated serum immunoglobulin G4 (IgG4) levels. About 10% of patients with PSC have elevated serum IgG4 levels. Unlike patients with classic PSC, patients with IgG4-associated disease usually respond to corticosteroids.

G. High-dose (>28 mg/kg/day) ursodeoxycholic acid (UDCA) should not be used for the management of patients with PSC as it has been demonstrated to worsen the outcome compared to placebo. On the other hand, some placebo-controlled studies have shown that standard to intermediate-dose UDCA (13–23 mg/kg/day) may improve serum levels of ALP and bilirubin without any difference in mortality, progression to cirrhosis, or liver transplant. If UDCA is started, then biochemical response should be assessed at 6 months. If there is biochemical response (e.g., >50% decrease in ALP from baseline), then UDCA is continued. Otherwise, UDCA should be discontinued.

H. Patients with PSC should be screened for cholangiocarcinoma and gallbladder cancer (with cross-sectional imaging and CA-19-9 every 6–12 months) as well as colorectal cancer (with annual colonoscopy). In addition, screening for esophageal varices, osteoporosis, and fat-soluble vitamin deficiencies is an essential component of PSC management. Liver tests should be monitored every 3–4 months for early evidence of strictures or tumors.

I. Patients with PSC and decompensated cirrhosis should be referred for liver transplantation when their Model for End-Stage Liver Disease (MELD) score exceeds 14. Other indications for liver transplantation in PSC include recurrent cholangitis, cholangiocarcinoma (<3 cm in diameter, without metastasis), and intractable pruritus.

BIBLIOGRAPHY

1. Cynthia Levy, Christopher L. Bowlus. Primary and Secondary Sclerosing Cholangitis. Sleisenger and Fordtran's Gastrointestinal and Liver Disease. 11th ed. Elsevier; 2020.
2. Bowlus CL. Primary Sclerosing Cholangitis. Handbook of Liver Disease. Elsevier; 2017. 4th ed.
3. Bowlus C, Assis DN, Goldberg DS. Primary and Secondary Sclerosing Cholangitis. Zakim and Boyer's Hepatology. Elsevier; 2016. 7th ed.
4. Lindor KD, Kowdley KV, Harrison ME. American College of Gastroenterology. ACG clinical guideline: primary sclerosing cholangitis. *Am J Gastroenterol.* 2015;110(5):646–659.
5. Hartl L, Haslinger K, Angerer M, et al. Progressive cholestasis and associated sclerosing cholangitis are frequent complications of COVID-19 in patients with chronic liver disease. *Hepatology.* 2022;76(6):1563–1575. https://doi.org/10.1002/hep.32582.

ALGORITHM 35.1 Flowchart for the diagnosis and management of PSC. *ALP,* Alkaline phosphatase; *AMA,* antimitochondrial antibody; *ERCP,* endoscopic retrograde cholangiopancreatography; *IgG4,* immunoglobulin G4; *MRCP,* magnetic resonance cholangiopancreatography; *PSC,* primary sclerosing cholangitis; *UDCA,* ursodeoxycholic acid; *ULN,* upper limit of normal; *US,* ultrasound.

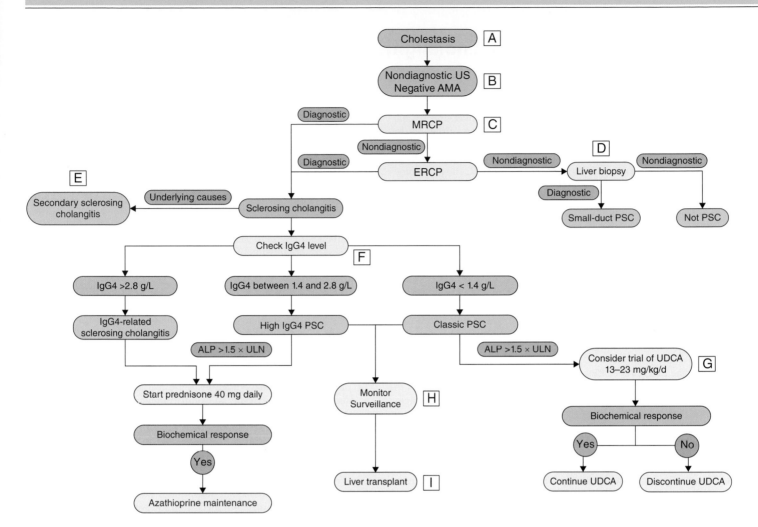

36 Primary Biliary Cholangitis

Emad Qayed

Primary biliary cholangitis (PBC) is an autoimmune liver disease characterized by inflammation and progressive destruction of the intrahepatic bile ducts. PBC is the most common chronic cholestatic liver disease in adults in the United States. It usually affects women between ages 40 and 60 years, with a female-to-male ratio of 9:1. PBC most commonly presents with fatigue and cholestasis (jaundice, itching), and it may progress to cirrhosis and portal hypertension. The disease is associated with several other autoimmune disorders such as Sjögren's syndrome, rheumatoid arthritis, CREST syndrome (Calcinosis cutis, Raynaud's phenomenon, Esophageal dysmotility, Sclerodactyly, and Telangiectasia), celiac disease, thyroiditis, interstitial nephritis, and skin disorders (lichen planus, discoid lupus, pemphigoid). The diagnosis of PBC is established when two out of three of the following criteria are met: (1) chronic cholestasis (alkaline phosphatase [ALKP] ≥1.5 times the upper limit of normal), (2) elevated serum antimitochondrial antibody or PBC specific antibodies such as anti-gp210 and anti-Sp100, and (3) liver histology consistent with PBC, revealing nonsuppurative destructive cholangitis with injury to the interlobular bile ducts.

A. Once the diagnosis of PBC is established, the presence of cirrhosis and clinical decompensation should be determined by reviewing the history, physical exam, and relevant laboratory and liver imaging tests. Patients with pruritus should be treated with cholestyramine, rifampicin, naltrexone, or sertraline. All patients should be evaluated for bone disease by a bone density study and prescribed vitamin D and calcium.

B. If cirrhosis is present, the patient should undergo hepatocellular carcinoma screening and upper endoscopy to screen for varices. Treatment options are limited in patients with hepatic decompensation or portal hypertension (Child-Pugh Class B or C grade, current or prior encephalopathy, ascites, esophageal or gastric varices). Therefore, treatment with ursodeoxycholic acid (UDCA) and referral to hepatology expert and transplant center are appropriate.

C. The first-line treatment for PBC is UDCA at 13–15 mg/kg/day, divided two to three times daily. Laboratory monitoring of ALKP, alanine transaminase (ALT), aspartate transaminase (AST), and bilirubin should be performed every 3–6 months while on therapy. UDCA should be discontinued in patients who are intolerant to the drug, and treatment with alternative agents such as obeticholic acid (OCA) or fenofibrates should be considered.

D. Patients who have adequate response to UDCA (decrease in ALKP to <1.5 upper limit of normal, and normal bilirubin) can continue maintenance therapy and laboratory monitoring.

E. Patients who have inadequate response to UDCA should be evaluated for autoimmune hepatitis-PBC overlap syndrome, and other causes of elevated liver enzymes and bilirubin should be considered (nonalcoholic steatohepatitis, occult celiac disease). It is important to ensure adequate UDCA dosing (13–15 mg/kg/day) and to confirm patient adherence to therapy. At this juncture, it is appropriate to reassess for progression of disease and development of decompensated cirrhosis.

F. In patients with decompensated cirrhosis and inadequate response to UDCA despite adequate dosing and adherence to therapy, referral to an expert/transplant center is reasonable. Based on the American Association for the Study of Liver Diseases (AASLD) updated practice guidance, OCA is contraindicated in decompensated cirrhosis and fenofibrates are discouraged in this patient population.

G. In patients with inadequate response to therapy who do not have decompensated cirrhosis, add-on treatment with OCA or fibrates is appropriate. OCA is started at a dose of 5 mg/day. If there is inadequate response at 6 months, then the dose is increased to 10 mg/day. Close monitoring is recommended in patients with cirrhosis. Fibrates (bezafibrate or fenofibrate) are an optional off-label alternative to OCA. They are preferred in patients with pruritus.

H. In patients with inadequate response to OCA or fibrates, the medication should be discontinued. Therapy with the alternative drug (OCA or fibrates) should be considered, and referral to hepatology expert and transplant center is appropriate.

BIBLIOGRAPHY

1. Sleisenger and Fordtran's Gastrointestinal and Liver Disease, 11th Edition, Elsevier, 2021. Chapter 91: Primary Biliary Cholangitis.
2. Lindor KD, Bowlus CL, Boyer J, Levy C, Mayo M. Primary biliary cholangitis: 2021 practice guidance update from the American Association for the Study of Liver Diseases. Hepatology. 2022;75(4):1012-1013. https://doi.org/10.1002/hep.32117

ALGORITHM 36.1 Flowchart for the management of primary biliary cholangitis *(PBC)*. *ALKP*, Alkaline phosphatase; *CBC*, complete blood count; *HCC*, hepatocellular carcinoma; *NASH*, nonalcoholic steatohepatitis; *OCA*, obeticholic acid; *UDCA*, ursodeoxycholic acid; *ULN*, upper limit of normal.

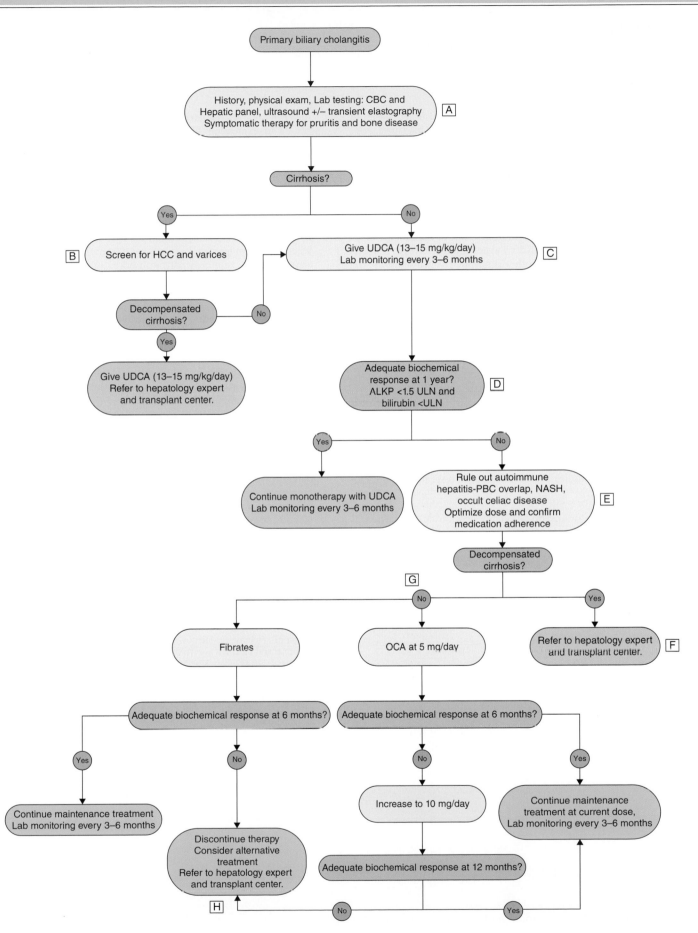

37 Hemochromatosis

Nikrad Shahnavaz

Hereditary hemochromatosis (HH) is an inherited disorder caused by impaired regulation of iron absorption from the small intestines, leading to iron overload and iron-mediated organ injury later in life. Classic HH (type 1) is most associated with autosomal recessive inheritance of mutations in the *HFE gene*. This mutation leads to altered function of the HFE protein, increased intestinal iron absorption due to reduced expression of the iron regulatory protein hepcidin. Most symptomatic patients with HFE-related HH are diagnosed between 40 and 50 years of age. C282Y homozygosity is equally frequent in men and women; however, it is more clinically apparent in men due to the iron loss from normal menstruation and childbirth in women. Other rare types of HH are associated with mutations in other genes such as hemojuvelin (HH type 2 A), hepcidin (HH type 2B), transferrin receptor 2 (HH type 3), and ferroportin (HH type 4).

A. The diagnosis of HH is suspected in patients with elevated serum aminotransferase levels, elevated iron stores, degenerative arthropathy, unexplained hepatomegaly, or unexplained hypogonadism. Other manifestations include skin hyperpigmentation, diabetes mellitus, heart failure, or amenorrhea.

B. The serum transferrin saturation and ferritin levels are the first tests to order when HH is suspected. However, the serum transferrin saturation is more sensitive and specific than the serum ferritin level as serum ferritin can be elevated in inflammatory conditions and other chronic liver diseases like nonalcoholic steatohepatitis (NASH). Transferrin saturation should be measured during fasting state to minimize the circadian and postprandial variations of its level.

C. Normal transferrin saturation level (<45%) will rule out classic HH (type 1), which accounts for more than 95% of patients with clinically expressed HH.

D. Elevation of the serum ferritin (in the absence of inflammatory conditions) associated with normal transferrin saturation can be seen in type 4 HH (ferroportin-related iron overload), a rare condition that is found in non-White patients. Liver biopsy is indicated to rule out this condition in patients with elevated liver enzymes and isolated elevation of ferritin levels.

E. Genetic testing for *HFE mutation* should be performed in all patients with elevated transferrin saturation, especially when associated with elevation of serum ferritin level. Genetic tests for non-HFE hemochromatosis are not currently available for clinical use.

F. Mutation of C282Y accounts for approximately 85%–90% of individuals with HH. Homozygosity for H63D, another mutation of the *HFE gene*, is associated with less severe iron overload and rarely results in expression of the clinical phenotype of HH. C282Y/H63D compound heterozygosity accounts for 5%–7% of clinically expressed HH.

G. There are two main indications for liver biopsy in patients being evaluated for HH: (1) for diagnosis of non-HFE HH in patients with elevated transferrin saturation or serum ferritin when HFE genotyping is negative and (2) for detecting the presence or absence of cirrhosis in a patient with classic HH when the liver enzymes are elevated, or when the serum ferritin level is above 1000 µg/L. Perls' Prussian blue stain is used to examine hepatic iron stores. In HFE-related HH, iron is typically found in periportal hepatocytes, and not in Kupffer cells. Symptomatic patients with HFE-related HH have a hepatic iron concentration (HIC) >10,000 µg/g dry weight (normal <1500 µg/g). In young and asymptomatic patients with early HFE-related HH, HIC is often less than 10,000 µg/g. MRI is another modality to diagnose cirrhosis and estimate hepatic liver content.

H. In patients with confirmed classic HH who have normal liver enzymes and serum ferritin is below 1000 µg/L, liver biopsy is not necessary. Phlebotomy is the treatment of choice. Phlebotomy can improve the survival if it is initiated before the development of cirrhosis. Phlebotomy of 500 mL (one unit) of whole blood is performed weekly, and the transferrin saturation and ferritin levels are checked at 2- to 3-month intervals. When ferritin level reaches between 50 and 100 ng/mL and transferrin saturation <50%, then iron stores are depleted, and management should proceed with maintenance phlebotomy of one unit of whole blood every 2–3 months. The goal is to keep transferrin saturation below 50% and ferritin level between 50 and 100 ng/mL. Phlebotomy should be paused if the hematocrit value drops below 37%. In patients who cannot tolerate phlebotomy due to anemia or congestive heart failure, chelating agents could be used as alternative treatment. Examples of chelating agents in HH include deferoxamine (given continuous subcutaneous infusion) and deferasirox (given as once-daily oral pill).

BIBLIOGRAPHY

1. Bacon BR, Fleming RE Hemochromatosis. Sleisenger and Fordtran's Gastrointestinal and Liver Disease. 11th Edition, Elsevier, 2020.
2. Procaccini NJ, Kowdley KV Hemochromatosis. Handbook of Liver Disease. 4th Edition, Elsevier, 2017.
3. Pietrangelo A Hemochromatosis. Zakim and Boyer's Hepatology. 7th Edition, Elsevier, 2018.
4. Qayed E Gastroenterology Clinical Focus: High yield GI and hepatology review- for Boards and Practice. 3rd Edition, Independently published. 2022.

ALGORITHM 37.1 Diagnostic approach for hereditary hemochromatosis *(HH)*.

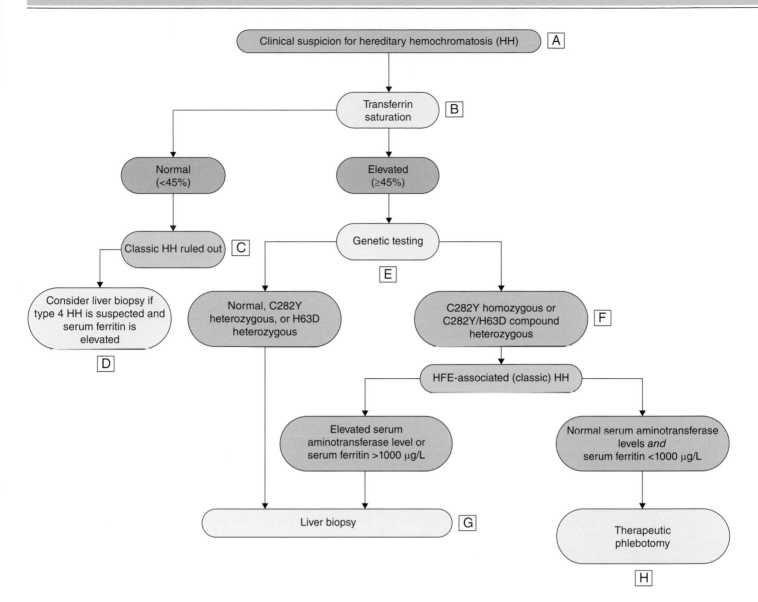

Clinical suspicion for hereditary hemochromatosis (HH) — A

Transferrin saturation — B

Normal (<45%)

Elevated (≥45%)

Classic HH ruled out — C

Genetic testing — E

Consider liver biopsy if type 4 HH is suspected and serum ferritin is elevated — D

Normal, C282Y heterozygous, or H63D heterozygous

C282Y homozygous or C282Y/H63D compound heterozygous — F

HFE-associated (classic) HH

Elevated serum aminotransferase level or serum ferritin >1000 µg/L

Normal serum aminotransferase levels *and* serum ferritin <1000 µg/L

Liver biopsy — G

Therapeutic phlebotomy — H

38 Wilson Disease

Emad Qayed

Wilson disease is an autosomal recessive disorder of copper metabolism that leads to copper accumulation in various organs such as the liver, brain, and cornea. It is caused by a defect in the ATP7B gene, which encodes a copper-transporting P-type adenosine triphosphatase (ATPase) involved in the transmembrane transport of copper and is expressed mainly in the hepatocytes.

Most patients with symptomatic Wilson disease present with liver disease in the second or third decades of life, or with neuropsychiatric features in the third or fourth decade of life. Wilson disease can lead to asymptomatic elevation of liver enzymes, hepatic steatosis, chronic hepatitis, cirrhosis, acute rapidly progressive hepatitis, or acute liver failure. It can also present as progressive neurologic disease without clinically significant hepatitis, acute hemolysis, or psychiatric illness (depression, bipolar disorder, neurotic behavior, psychosis). The diagnosis of Wilson disease requires the presence of clinical signs and biochemical tests, or the detection of disease-specific mutations of ATP7B by molecular testing. The main treatment options for Wilson disease are dietary restriction of copper, D-penicillamine, trientine, and zinc. D-Penicillamine and trientine are general chelators that stimulate excretion of copper in urine, while zinc blocks intestinal copper absorption.

A. Wilson disease should be considered in persons with:
- Unexplained elevations of serum aminotransferases, chronic hepatitis with steatosis, autoimmune hepatitis that is poorly responsive to therapy, unexplained cirrhosis, or acute liver failure. Acute liver failure due to Wilson disease has a characteristic clinical presentation which includes acute Coombs-negative hemolysis leading to severe drop in hemoglobin, renal failure, low aminotransferase levels, normal or low alkaline phosphatase level, and elevated total bilirubin level (unconjugated hyperbilirubinemia). The ratio of alkaline phosphatase to total bilirubin is less than 4 and the ratio of alanine transaminase (ALT) to aspartate transaminase (AST) is greater than 2.2.
- Neurologic features of unexplained origin (abnormal behavior, incoordination, dysarthria, tremor, dyskinesia, or rigid dystonia).
- A neurologic or psychiatric disorder combined with signs of hepatic disease.
- Presence of Kayser-Fleischer (KF) rings. These rings represent copper deposition in Descemet's membrane of the cornea, and are seen in slit-lamp ophthalmologic examination. Other ocular manifestations of Wilson disease include sunflower cataracts, which are deposits of copper in the lens.
- Unexplained, acquired Coombs-negative hemolytic anemia.
- A first-degree relative with Wilson disease.

B. The workup for suspected Wilson disease includes history, physical examination (focused on the liver, neurologic, and psychiatric evaluation), ophthalmologic slit-lamp examination, complete blood count, international normalized ratio (INR), liver panel, serum ceruloplasmin, and 24-hour urinary excretion of copper.

C. If KF rings are present, ceruloplasmin <20 mg/dL, and 24-hour urinary copper excretion is >40 μg, this is consistent with Wilson disease.

D. If KF rings are absent, ceruloplasmin <20 mg/dL, and 24-hour urinary copper excretion is >100 μg, this is consistent with Wilson disease.

E. If KF rings are absent, ceruloplasmin ≥20 mg/dL, and 24-hour urinary copper ≤40 μg, this excludes Wilson disease.

F. Liver biopsy with copper quantification should be considered for all other scenarios in which liver disease is present and Wilson disease is suspected, but initial tests do not confirm nor exclude the diagnosis. If hepatic copper concentration is >250 μg/g, this is consistent with Wilson disease. If there is a low suspicion of Wilson disease, a copper content of <50 μg/g excludes the diagnosis of Wilson disease. Liver biopsy also provides information about the grade and stage of liver injury, the degree of fibrosis, and helps to exclude other liver diseases.

G. If liver biopsy and copper quantification do not confirm the diagnosis of Wilson disease, molecular genetic testing of *ATP7B* gene should be performed. If pathogenic gene variants are found on both alleles, this confirms Wilson disease.

BIBLIOGRAPHY

1. Handbook of Liver Disease, Chapter 19. Wilson Disease and Related Disorders. Elsevier, 2018.
2. Schilsky ML, Roberts EA, Bronstein JM, et al. A multidisciplinary approach to the diagnosis and management of Wilson disease: 2022 practice guidance on Wilson disease from the American Association for the Study of Liver Diseases. *Hepatology*. Published online December 7, 2022. https://doi.org/10.1002/hep.32801.
3. Sleisenger and Fordtran's Gastrointestinal and Liver Disease, 11th Edition, Elsevier, 2021. Chapter 76: Wilson disease.

ALGORITHM 38.1 Flowchart for the workup of suspected Wilson disease. *Cu*, Copper; *KF*, Kayser-Fleischer.

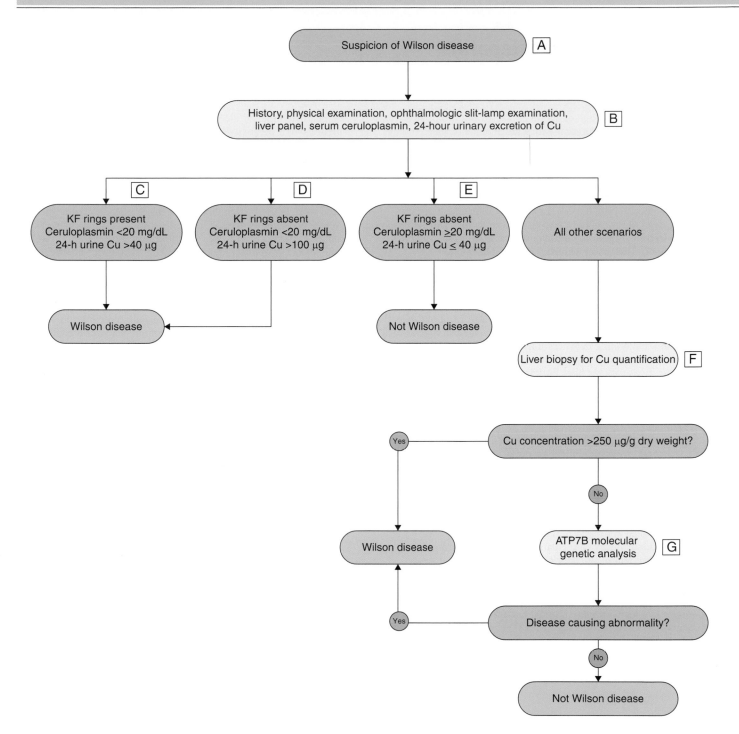

39 Alcoholic Hepatitis

Elnaz Jafarimehr

Alcoholic liver disease is one of the main causes of chronic liver disease worldwide, and it can present with a range of histological findings, including steatosis, steatohepatitis, and fibrosis. Symptomatic steatohepatitis or cirrhosis can present acutely as acute alcoholic hepatitis, which is associated with high morbidity and mortality.

A. There are clinical diagnostic criteria for alcoholic hepatitis in patients with history of alcohol use disorder, which include:
   1. History of heavy alcohol use: >40 g/day in women and >60 g/day in men for a minimum period of 6 months.
   2. Alcohol consumption within 60 days of presentation.
   3. Bilirubin levels >3 mg/dL; an aspartate transaminase (AST)/ alanine transaminase (ALT) ratio of >1.5, with the levels of each between 50 IU/L and 400 IU/L.

Using clinical diagnostic criteria and liver biopsy, we categorize patients to have definite, possible, or probable alcoholic hepatitis. Liver biopsy usually shows centrilobular and perivenular fatty infiltration, ballooning degeneration of hepatocytes, alcoholic hyaline (Mallory, or Mallory-Denk, bodies), and neutrophilic infiltrates. The majority of patients have fatty infiltration and varying degrees of fibrosis.

B. The severity of the disease is assessed by calculating the Maddrey's Discrimination Function (MDF) or Model for End-Stage Liver Disease (MELD) score. MDF: {[4.6 × prothrombin time − control value (seconds)] + serum bilirubin (mg/dL)}.

C. If MDF >32 or MELD >20 then prednisolone 40 mg daily is started, if there are no contraindication for starting prednisolone, which includes:
   - Uncontrolled infection.
   - Uncontrolled upper gastrointestinal (GI) bleeding.
   - Acute kidney injury with creatinine more than 2.5 mg/dL.
   - Multiorgan failure and shock.
   - Concomitant infection including hepatitis B and C, HIV, tuberculosis (TB), acute pancreatitis, drug-induced liver injury (DILI), and hepatocellular carcinoma (HCC).

Conservative management and nutritional support is considered in patients who do not have a high MELD or MDF score. The steroids or pentoxifylline for alcoholic hepatitis (STOPAH) trial evaluated prednisolone, pentoxifylline, and placebo in severe alcoholic hepatitis. There was a modest beneficial effect of prednisolone on mortality at 28 days, but no beneficial effect beyond 28 days. The overall 1-year mortality rate was 56%. The study found no impact of pentoxifylline on survival.

D. Lille score is used to predict treatment response to corticosteroids in patients beyond 7 days. Lille model score incorporates age, serum albumin, serum creatinine, prothrombin time, serum bilirubin, and change in bilirubin level at day 7. Patients with a score ≥ 0.45 have a 6-month survival rate of 25%, and glucocorticoids can be discontinued.

E. Early transplant has survival benefit for patients who are not responding to corticosteroids based on Lille score but only a small percentage of patients with severe alcoholic hepatitis are eligible to early liver transplantation. Novel therapies are emerging to salvage patients with alcoholic hepatitis. There are multiple clinical trials investigating the effect of the medication that modulate the gut-liver axis, agents with antiinflammatory activity, antioxidant activity, and antiregenerative activity.

BIBLIOGRAPHY

1. Han MAT, Pyrsopoulos N, Emerging therapies for alcoholic hepatitis. *Clin Liver Dis.* 2021;25(3):603-624.
2. Singal AK, Bataller R, Ahn J, et al. ACG clinical guideline: alcoholic liver disease. *Am J Gastroenterol.* 2018;113(2):175-194.
3. Sehrawat TS, Liu M, Shah VH. The knowns and unknowns of treatment for alcoholic hepatitis. *Lancet Gastroenterol Hepatol.* 2020;5(5):494-506.
4. Crabb DW, Im GY, Szabo G, Mellinger JL, Lucey MR. Diagnosis and treatment of alcohol-associated liver diseases: 2019 practice guidance from the American Association for the Study of Liver Diseases. *Hepatology.* 2020;71(1):306-333.
5. Forrest E, Mellor J, Stanton L Steroids or pentoxifylline for alcoholic hepatitis (STOPAH): study protocol for a randomised controlled trial. *Trials.* 2013;14:262. https://doi.org/10.1186/1745-6215-14-262.
6. Szabo G, McClain CJ Alcohol-associated liver disease. Sleisenger and Fordtran's Gastrointestinal and Liver Disease. 11th Edition, Elsevier, 2020.

ALGORITHM 39.1 Flowchart for the diagnosis and management of acute alcoholic hepatitis. Model for End-Stage Liver Disease *(MELD)* for end-stage liver disease.

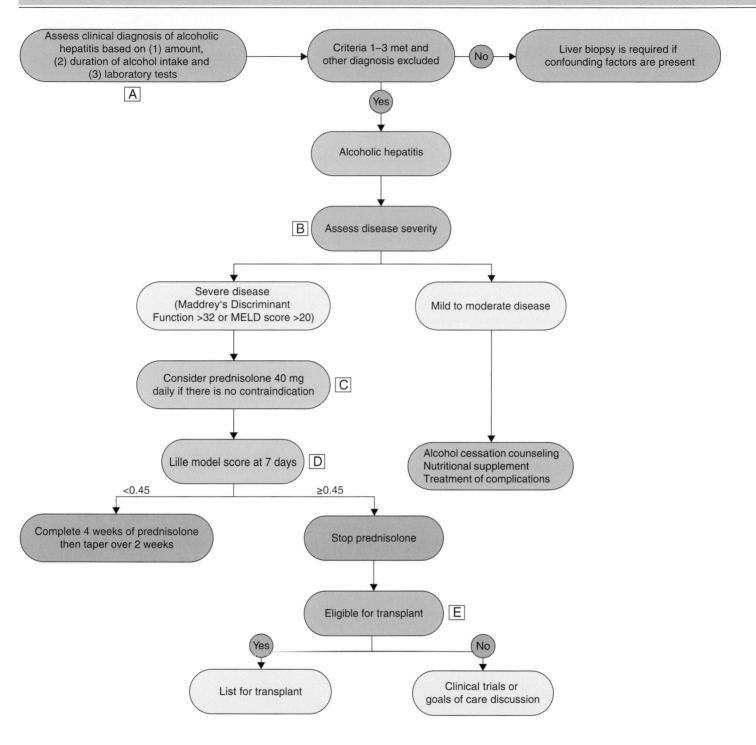

40 Autoimmune Hepatitis

Emad Qayed

Autoimmune hepatitis (AIH) is a chronic inflammatory disease of the liver characterized by the presence of interface hepatitis on histology, circulating autoantibodies, and hypergammaglobulinemia. Asymptomatic patients with AIH present with elevated transaminase levels, while symptomatic patients can present with acute hepatitis, acute liver failure, or chronic hepatitis and cirrhosis. The diagnosis of AIH relies on the presence of a constellation of clinical, laboratory, and histologic findings such as positive autoantibodies (e.g., anti-nuclear antibody [ANA], smooth muscle antibody [SMA], and anti-LKM1 antibody), elevated γ-globulin levels, and characteristic histologic findings of interface hepatitis. Interface hepatitis (previously referred to as piecemeal necrosis) is characterized by dense, plasma cell–rich inflammation in the hepatic parenchyma at its junction with the portal tracts. This finding is present in up to 98% of patients with AIH.

A. The initial evaluation of a patient with features of AIH requires careful review of the history, physical exam, and laboratory and histologic workup. The differential diagnosis of AIH includes Wilson disease, chronic viral hepatitis, non-alcoholic fatty liver disease (NAFLD), overlap syndromes (AIH-primary sclerosing cholangitis, AIH-primary biliary cholangitis) and drug-induced AIH. The majority of patients with drug-induced AIH are women who develop acute elevation of liver enzymes, and may present with fevers, rash, and eosinophilia. Drugs that have been definitely associated with AIH include minocycline, nitrofurantoin, anti-tumor necrosis factor (TNF) agents, methyldopa, and halothane. Other associated drugs include those with probable association with AIH (diclofenac, propylthiouracil, atorvastatin, rosuvastatin, isoniazid) and possible association (indomethacin, clometacin, immune checkpoint inhibitors). Patients with newly diagnosed AIH should be screened for autoimmune thyroid disease and celiac disease.

B. The presence of cirrhosis should be determined based on clinical, radiologic, and histologic findings. Cirrhosis is present in approximately one-third of patients at presentation, and it is more common in patients older than 60 years.

C. In patients without cirrhosis, the first-line therapy is combination prednisone (or prednisolone) and azathioprine. An alternative to prednisone is budesonide.

D. In patients with compensated cirrhosis, the first-line therapy is combination prednisone (or prednisolone) and azathioprine; budesonide should not be used. Avoid azathioprine in patients with decompensated cirrhosis.

E. Laboratory monitoring of transaminase levels is performed every 2 weeks, and treatment response is assessed at 4–8 weeks.

F. In patients who respond to treatment, prednisone and budesonide should be slowly tapered and azathioprine continued (if started).

G. If transaminase and immunoglobulin levels normalize at 6 months, this establishes biochemical remission. In patients on combination therapy with steroids and azathioprine, consider complete steroid withdrawal, and perform lab testing every 3–4 months.

H. If prolonged biochemical remission is achieved in which transaminase levels are normal at 24 months, consider treatment discontinuation and close monitoring for relapse. Performing a liver biopsy to confirm complete histologic remission is optional prior to treatment discontinuation. In patients who are tolerating treatment and would like to avoid the possibility of relapse, it is appropriate to continue treatment without attempting treatment discontinuation.

I. In patients who do not respond to initial treatment and have worsening liver transaminase level (treatment failure) or respond but do not achieve biochemical remission at 6 months (incomplete response), second-line therapies should be considered. These include high-dose steroids and azathioprine (if not already given), mycophenolate mofetil, tacrolimus, and cyclosporine.

BIBLIOGRAPHY

1. Mack CL, Adams D, Assis DN, et al. Diagnosis and management of autoimmune hepatitis in adults and children: 2019 practice guidance and guidelines from the American Association for the Study of Liver Diseases. *Hepatology.* 2020;72(2):671-722. https://doi.org/10.1002/hep.31065.
2. Sleisenger and Fordtran's. Gastrointestinal and Liver Disease, 11th Edition, Elsevier, 2020. Chapter 90: Autoimmune hepatitis.
3. Muratori L, Lohse AW, Lenzi M. Diagnosis and management of autoimmune hepatitis [published correction appears in BMJ. 2023;380:p330]. *BMJ.* 2023;380:e070201. Published 2023 Feb 6. https://doi.org/10.1136/bmj-2022-070201.

ALGORITHM 40.1 Flowchart for the initial workup and management of autoimmune hepatitis *(AIH).* Treatment of acute severe hepatitis and acute liver failure due to AIH is not discussed in this algorithm. These severe presentations require high-dose steroids and urgent liver transplant evaluation. *ALT,* Alanine transaminase; *AST,* aspartate transaminase; *CBC,* complete blood count; *HCC,* hepatocellular carcinoma; *IgG,* immunoglobulin G; *PBC,* primary biliary cirrhosis; *PSC,* primary sclerosing cholangitis; *TPMT,* thiopurine methyltransferase.

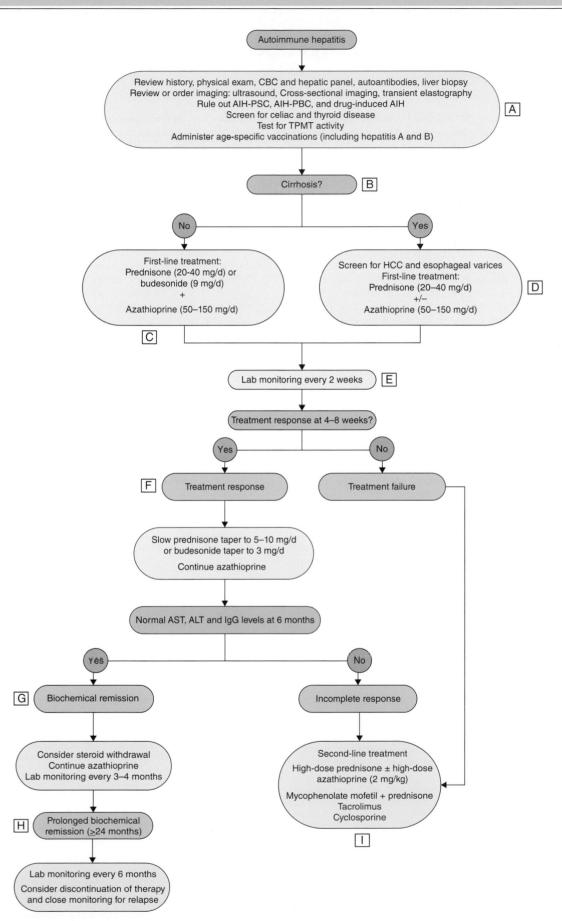

41 Nonalcoholic Fatty Liver Disease

Thuy-Van Pham Hang

Nonalcoholic fatty liver disease (NAFLD) is a common disease affecting more than one-third of individuals in the United States. The American Association for the Study of Liver Disease defines NAFLD by the presence of the following four criteria: hepatic steatosis on imaging or histology, no significant alcohol consumption (typically defined as >21 standard drinks/week in men or >14 standard drinks/week for women), no competing causes of hepatic steatosis, and no coexisting causes of chronic liver diseases. Nonalcoholic steatohepatitis (NASH) is a progressive subtype of NAFLD characterized by inflammation, ballooning, and Mallory's hyaline on liver biopsy. NASH can lead to hepatic fibrosis, cirrhosis, and hepatocellular cancer (HCC). In general, patients with NASH have increased morbidity and mortality from cardiovascular disease, and advanced liver fibrosis is associated with increasing number of metabolic comorbidities. Groups at high risk for developing NASH-related fibrosis include those with type 2 diabetes mellitus (DM), ≥2 metabolic risk factors (central obesity, dyslipidemia, hypertension, prediabetes, insulin resistance), and those with elevated aminotransferases.

A. It is important to rule out other etiologies of liver disease. A thorough clinical assessment should focus on evaluating for metabolic comorbidities and quantifying alcohol consumption. Laboratory workup includes complete blood count, complete metabolic panel, hepatitis B and C serologies, antinuclear antibodies (ANA), antimitochondrial antibodies (AMA), anti–smooth muscle antibodies (ASMA), immunoglobulins, ferritin, and alpha-1 antitrypsin (A1AT).

B. Fibrosis-4 (FIB-4) is a noninvasive test for fibrosis. It is a calculated value based on age, aspartate transaminase (AST), alanine transaminase (ALT), and platelet count. FIB-4 has excellent diagnostic accuracy for advanced fibrosis in NAFLD.

C. FIB-4 <1.3 (or <2 in those >65 years old) has a negative predictive value of ≥90% with regards to the presence of advanced fibrosis. Patients with low FIB-4 score require no further workup, and management is focused on keeping a healthy lifestyle and treatment of any metabolic comorbidities. Repeat noninvasive testing with fibrosis score in 2–3 years.

D. Patients with an intermediate risk of advanced fibrosis should undergo liver stiffness measurement, as determined by vibration-controlled transient elastography (e.g., FibroScan). The kilopascal (kPA) cutoffs used in this algorithm are based on the American Gastroenterological Association's 2022 clinical care pathway for risk stratification of patients with NAFLD.

E. Patients with intermediate risk of advanced fibrosis based on liver stiffness measurement should be referred to a hepatologist with consideration of further workup (magnetic resonance elastography), monitoring, or liver biopsy to confirm fibrosis staging and steatohepatitis.

F. Patients with high FIB-4 scores or those with high liver stiffness measurements should be referred to a hepatologist. Further workup includes liver stiffness measurement (if not already performed) and liver biopsy to confirm the presence of steatohepatitis and level of fibrosis. Patients with advanced fibrosis from NASH are at risk of developing HCC and should receive screening with ultrasound (with or without alpha-fetoprotein) every 6 months.

G. In patients with NASH, weight loss >5% total body weight decreases hepatic steatosis, while weight loss >7% can lead to resolution of NASH and weight loss >10% can result in fibrosis regression or stability. Clinically significant weight loss requires a hypocaloric diet (1200–1500 kcal daily or reduction from baseline of 500–1000 kcal daily). A hypocaloric diet is also recommended in patients with lean NASH (body mass index <25 kg/m² for non-Asians or body mass index <23 kg/m² in Asians); however, in this population, a lower weight loss target of 3%–5% body weight leads to similar histologic benefits to those with NASH who are overweight or obese. In general, the Mediterranean diet is recommended. Select patients may benefit from antiobesity medications and bariatric surgery. Regarding exercise, 150–300 minutes of moderate-intensity exercise (3–6 metabolic equivalents) or 75–100 minutes of vigorous-intensity exercise per week is recommended.

H. There are no medications currently approved by the US Food and Drug Administration for the treatment of NASH. In patients with concurrent DM, pioglitazone (a thiazolidinedione) and glucagon-like peptide-1 receptor agonists (GLP-1RAs) such as liraglutide and semaglutide are the preferred treatment given demonstration of histologic improvement. Pioglitazone can lead to weight gain and is contraindicated in decompensated cirrhosis. GLP-1RAs can have dose-dependent gastrointestinal side effects. In patients with NASH without DM, vitamin E 800 IU daily can be considered as it can improve steatohepatitis in this population. Of note, vitamin E 400 IU daily has been associated with an increased risk of prostate cancer.

BIBLIOGRAPHY

1. Ando Y, Jou JH. Nonalcoholic fatty liver disease and recent guideline updates. *Clin Liver Dis (Hoboken)*. 2021;17(1):23-28.
2. Chalasani N, Younossi Z, Lavine JE, et al. The diagnosis and management of nonalcoholic fatty liver disease: practice guidance from the American Association for the Study of Liver Diseases. *Hepatology*. 2018;67(1):328-357.
3. Kanwal F, Shubrook JH, Adams LA, et al. Clinical care pathway for the risk stratification and management of patients with nonalcoholic fatty liver disease. *Gastroenterology*. 2021;161(5):1657-1669.
4. Long MT, Noureddin M, Lim JK. AGA clinical practice update: diagnosis and management of nonalcoholic fatty liver disease in lean individuals: expert review. *Gastroenterology*. 2022;163(3):764-774.e1.
5. Younossi ZM, Corey KE, Lim JK. AGA clinical practice update on lifestyle modification using diet and exercise to achieve weight loss in the management of nonalcoholic fatty liver disease: expert review. *Gastroenterology*. 2021;160(3):912-918.

ALGORITHM 41.1 Flowchart of the diagnosis and management of nonalcoholic fatty liver disease *(NAFLD)*. *FIB-4*, Fibrosis-4; *GLP1-RA*, glucagon-like peptide-1 receptor agonist; *MRE*, magnetic resonance elastography.

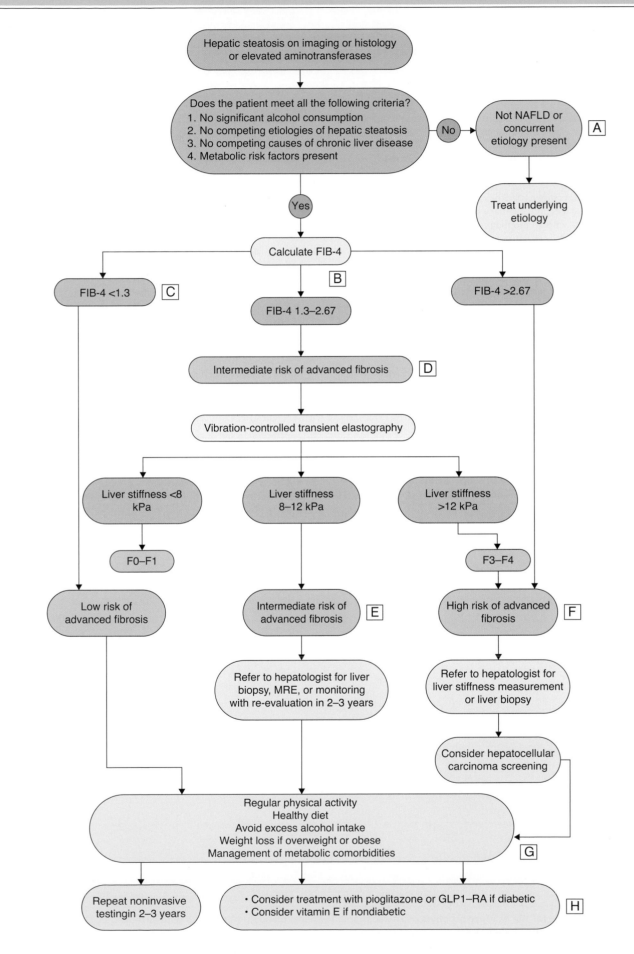

Prophylaxis of Esophageal Variceal Bleeding

Emad Qayed

Prevention of esophageal variceal bleeding is an important management piece in the comprehensive care of patients with cirrhosis. Patients who experienced prior esophageal variceal bleeding should undergo both esophageal ligation and receive nonselective beta-blockers (NSBBs), unless they previously had portosystemic shunt placement.

A. In patients with decompensated cirrhosis and no prior history of esophageal variceal bleeding, primary prophylaxis of esophageal variceal bleeding starts with an esophagogastroduodenoscopy (EGD) to evaluate for the presence of varices.

B. Patients with compensated cirrhosis can alternatively undergo noninvasive assessment of liver stiffness (transient elastography). If liver stiffness is <20 kPa and platelet count is >150,000/mm³, the chances of having significant varices on EGD are small, and EGD can be deferred. A repeat evaluation with the same tests is recommended in 1 year. If hepatic decompensation develops, a screening EGD is required.

C. If EGD is performed and there are no esophageal varices, repeat EGD in 2–3 years. Experts recommend that the interval should be 2 years if there is ongoing liver injury (e.g., active alcohol drinking, active hepatitis). Otherwise, a repeat EGD in 3 years is appropriate.

D. If esophageal varices are present, they should be described in terms of their location (lower third, middle third, and upper third of the esophagus), presence of red color signs, and the size of the varices. The red signs include red "wale" markings, cherry-red spots, or diffuse redness. Small varices are 5 mm or less in diameter, while large varices are greater than 5 mm in diameter. If there are small esophageal varices without high-risk stigmata, repeat EGD in 1–2 years. Consider 1-year interval if there is ongoing liver injury and 2 years in the absence of ongoing injury.

E. The American Association for the Study of Liver Diseases (AASLD) recommends NSBB if there are small esophageal varices with high-risk stigmata (e.g., red wale signs) or if they occur in patients with advanced cirrhosis.

F. If large varices are encountered, management should proceed with either NSBB or endoscopic variceal band ligation (EVL).

G. NSBB should be titrated to achieve a heart rate of 55–60 beats per minute. If this cannot be achieved or if the patient does not tolerate therapy, then NSBB should be discontinued and EVL should be performed.

H. EVL should be repeated every 2–8 weeks until complete eradication of varices is achieved, and then EGD should be repeated every 6–12 months for surveillance.

BIBLIOGRAPHY

1. Garcia-Tsao G, Abraldes JG, Berzigotti A, Bosch J. Portal hypertensive bleeding in cirrhosis: risk stratification, diagnosis, and management: 2016 practice guidance by the American Association for the study of liver diseases. *Hepatology*. 2017;65(1):310-335. Erratum in: Hepatology. 2017;66(1):304.
2. Sleisenger and Fordtran's Gastrointestinal and Liver Disease, 11th Edition, Elsevier, 2021. Chapter 92: Portal Hypertension and Variceal Bleeding.

ALGORITHM 42.1 Flowchart for the primary prophylaxis of esophageal variceal bleeding in patients with cirrhosis. *EGD*: Esophagogastroduodenoscopy; *NSBB*, nonselective beta blocker.

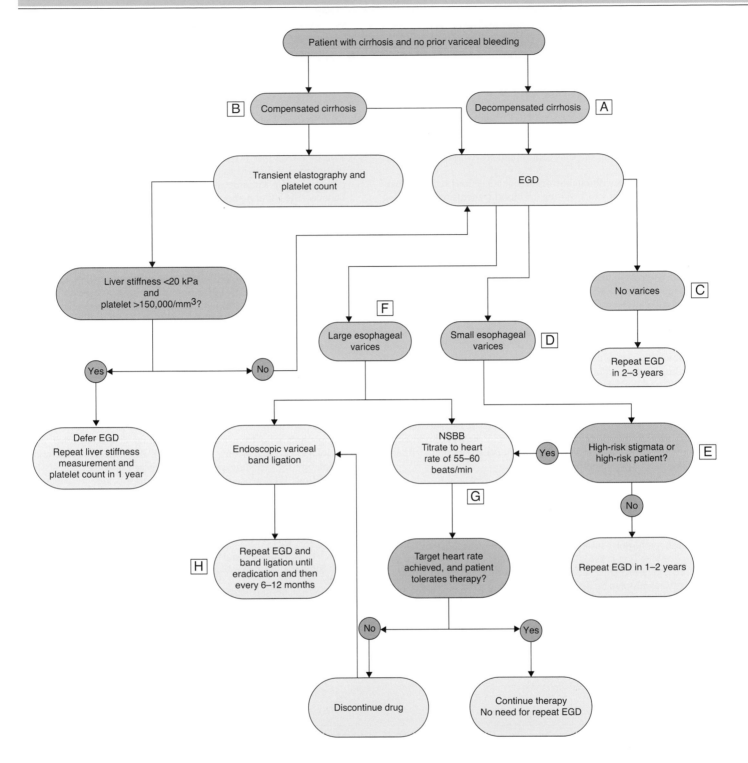

43 Esophageal Variceal Bleeding

Nikrad Shahnavaz

Acute esophageal variceal bleeding is a life-threatening emergency and requires management by an experienced multidisciplinary team of gastroenterologists, intensivists, and radiologists. The goal of the treatment is hemodynamic resuscitation, bleeding control, and prevention of rebleeding.

A. Resuscitation starts with establishing adequate venous access, initiating intravenous fluid while waiting for blood transfusion, protecting the airway in patients with massive bleeding or with hepatic encephalopathy, and inserting a nasogastric tube to assess the severity of bleeding and to lavage gastric contents before endoscopy. A restrictive strategy in which blood transfusion is given when the hemoglobin level drops below 7 g/dL is associated with improved outcomes. Vasoactive agents like octreotide, somatostatin, or terlipressin should be started as soon as possible in the emergency room when variceal bleeding is suspected. Octreotide is the most common vasoactive agent used in the United States and is given as an initial bolus of 50 mcg followed by continuous infusion of 50 mcg/h. It should be continued for 3–5 days after initiation of treatment. Administration of antibiotics upon presentation is important to reduce the risk of rebleeding and spontaneous bacterial peritonitis. Ceftriaxone (1 g every 24 hours) is the antibiotic of choice.

B. Endoscopic variceal ligation (EVL) is the preferred endoscopic therapy for acute bleeding from esophageal varices. It has success rates of 80%–90% in initial control of variceal hemorrhage. Endoscopic therapy is carried out as soon as the patient is hemodynamically stabilized, within 12 hours of hospital admission.

C. In patients who are high-risk for treatment failure (Child-Pugh class C, Child-Pugh class B with active bleeding, or model for end-stage liver disease (MELD) score >18 and requirement for transfusion of >4 units of red blood cells [RBCs]), the early use of transjugular intrahepatic portosystemic shunt (TIPS) within 72 hours of the control of bleeding is associated with reduced risk of mortality and treatment failure. After successful placement of TIPS, intravenous vasoactive agents can be discontinued. These patients do not require further therapy for secondary prophylaxis after discharge, but should be referred for liver transplant evaluation. TIPS patency should be assessed by Doppler ultrasound every 6 months at the time of hepatocellular carcinoma (HCC) screening.

D. In 10%–20% of cases in which pharmacologic and endoscopic therapy fail to control the variceal bleeding, balloon tamponade may be of value as a temporizing treatment before proceeding with more definitive treatment like TIPS. In most cases, inflation of the gastric balloon alone is sufficient to control the bleeding, thereby avoiding the potential complications associated with inflation of the esophageal balloon. The balloon should not be used for longer than 24 hours to reduce the risk of esophageal necrosis.

E. The risk of recurrent variceal bleeding is highest in the first few weeks to months after the index hemorrhage. Therefore it is critical that secondary prophylaxis be initiated as soon as the acute bleeding episode is controlled. Combination of endoscopic (EVL every 1–2 weeks after the index bleeding and until the varices are obliterated) and pharmacologic treatment (either nonselective beta-adrenergic blockers [NSBBs] including propranolol and nadolol, or carvedilol) is preferred for the prevention of recurrent variceal bleeding. The dosage of NSBBs should be titrated for the goal heart rate of 55–60 as long as systolic blood pressure remains above 90 mm Hg. Carvedilol should be avoided in patients with refractory ascites. Medical therapy is the cornerstone of combination therapy. Therefore, if patient cannot tolerate the drug despite dose adjustment, TIPS should be considered to prevent recurrent variceal bleeding.

F. For patients who have variceal rebleeding despite optimal pharmacologic and endoscopic treatment, TIPS is the preferred choice of therapy for reducing portal hypertension and therefore risk of rebleeding. TIPS procedure can be used as a bridge to liver transplantation in appropriate candidates.

BIBLIOGRAPHY

1. Shah VH, Kamath PS Portal hypertension and variceal bleeding. Sleisenger and Fordtran's Gastrointestinal and Liver Disease. 11th Edition, Elsevier, 2020.
2. Grace ND, Stoffel EM, Puleo J Portal hypertension and gastrointestinal bleeding. Handbook of Liver Disease. 4th Edition, Elsevier, 2017.
3. Garcia-Tsao G, Abraldes JG, Berzigotti A, Bosch J Portal hypertensive bleeding in cirrhosis: risk stratification, diagnosis, and management. Hepatology. 2017;65(1):310-335.

ALGORITHM 43.1 The management of bleeding esophageal varices and secondary prophylaxis. *EGD*, Esophagogastroduodenoscopy; *EVL*, endoscopic variceal ligation; *MELD*, model for end-stage liver disease; *RBC*, red blood cell; *TIPS*, transjugular intrahepatic portosystemic shunt.

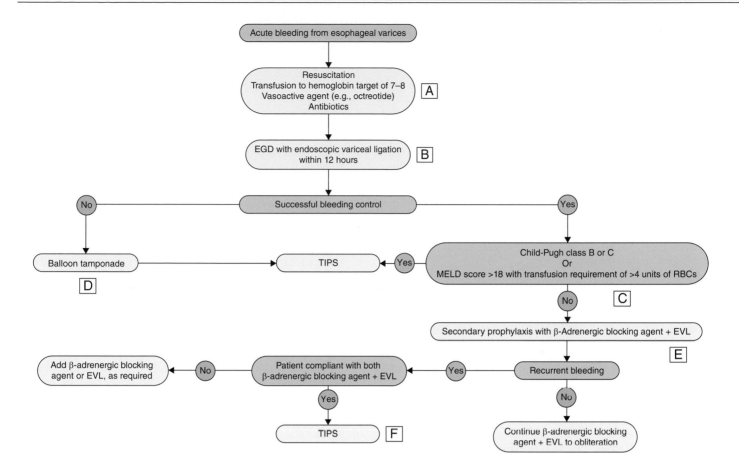

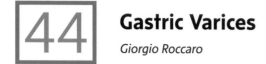

Gastric Varices

Giorgio Roccaro

Gastric varices are dilated portosystemic collateral blood vessels that develop due to portal hypertension or extrahepatic portal vein or splenic vein obstruction. The prevalence of gastric varices is estimated to be between 15% and 20% in patients with cirrhosis. They are often classified according to their location within the stomach. Varices in direct continuity with the esophagus along the lesser and greater curvatures of the stomach are called *gastroesophageal varices* (*GOV*) types 1 and 2, respectively. Isolated gastric varices (IGV) are classified as type I (IGV1) if they occur in the fundus and type 2 (IGV2) if they occur elsewhere. Risk of hemorrhage is greatest among those with IGV1. Acute hemorrhage from gastric varices is associated with higher mortality compared to esophageal varices bleeding.

A. Nonbleeding gastric varices are typically discovered during routine screening upper endoscopy. Nonselective beta-blocker (NSBB) therapy, such as propranolol or nadolol, is recommended for primary prophylaxis of acute variceal hemorrhage from gastric varices, especially GOV2 or IGV1 that have not bled. The primary prophylaxis of GOV1 is similar to that of esophageal varices. The data to support endoscopic therapy such as cyanoacrylate (CYA) glue injection for primary prophylaxis of gastric varices are lacking, although it may be performed in clinical practice for patients who cannot tolerate NSBBs.

B. In the setting of acute gastric variceal hemorrhage, the initial steps leading up to endoscopic diagnosis and targeted therapy are the same as in esophageal variceal hemorrhage. This includes admission to an intensive care unit for initial resuscitation with packed red blood cells transfusion targeting hemodynamic stability and a hemoglobin of approximately 8 g/dL, protection of the airway with endotracheal intubation, administration of empiric broad-spectrum antibiotics to decrease risk of bacterial infection associated with increased mortality, and infusion of vasoactive agents associated with splanchnic vasoconstriction such as octreotide, vasopressin, and terlipressin. Urgent upper endoscopy, once the patient has been stabilized, must be performed within 12 hours of presentation for diagnosis and treatment.

C. Data regarding the efficacy of endoscopic therapy for the treatment of bleeding gastric varices are limited; current available endoscopic interventions include endoscopic injection sclerotherapy (EIS), tissue adhesive injection such as CYA, and endoscopic variceal ligation (EVL). EIS with sclerosing agents such as alcohol, polidocanol, or tetradecyl sulfate is associated with increased complications and rebleeding and is thus not recommended.

D. CYA glue is a synthetic glue which rapidly polymerizes into a hard acrylic upon injection into a blood vessel. It is recommended for the treatment of acute bleeding from IGV and GOV2 varices, when

endoscopist is familiar with this technique. Otherwise, EVL is recommended, especially for small GOV2.

E. Acute hemorrhage from GOV1 can be treated with EVL similar to esophageal varices.

F. If acute gastric variceal bleeding is not amenable to be controlled with endoscopic intervention, then transjugular intrahepatic portosystemic shunt (TIPS) or balloon-occluded retrograde transvenous obliteration (BRTO) should be performed. TIPS is an invasive procedure that creates an intrahepatic connection between the hepatic and the portal venous system resulting in the diversion of the portal venous directly into systemic circulation, thereby reducing portal venous pressure. It is the treatment of choice in acute gastric variceal bleeding, especially GOV2 and IGV1. BRTO is an invasive technique that involves the retrograde injection of a sclerosing agent and metallic coils into gastric varices after occluding the portosystemic shunt with an occlusion balloon under fluoroscopic guidance. The performance of BRTO requires the presence of a spontaneous portosystemic shunt such as a gastro-renal shunt or a gastro-caval, which is present in 60%–85% of cases. This may be the approach of choice in patients with refractory hepatic encephalopathy, poor liver function, or complete portal vein thrombosis.

G. Given the effectiveness of minimally invasive techniques via endoscopy and interventional radiology, the role of surgery in managing acute gastric variceal bleeding is limited and should be considered a last resort when the aforementioned measures fail. However, splenectomy or splenic artery embolization should be considered a means of definitive therapy in patients with acute gastric variceal bleeding secondary to sinistral or left-sided portal hypertension caused by splenic vein thrombosis (SVT). Splenectomy eliminates collateral venous flow and prevents future gastric variceal bleeding secondary to SVT.

H. NSBBs in combination with endoscopy therapy (EVL or CYA injection) are recommended as first-line secondary prophylaxis to prevent rebleeding in patients who recover from GOV1 bleeding. TIPS or BRTO is indicated as first-line secondary prophylaxis in patients who recover from gastric variceal hemorrhage secondary to GOV2 or IGV1 type of gastric varices.

BIBLIOGRAPHY

1. Sleisenger and Fordtran's Gastrointestinal and Liver Disease, 11th Edition, 2020. Chapter 92, Portal hypertension and variceal bleeding.
2. Henry Z, Patel K, Patton H, Saad W. AGA clinical practice update on management of bleeding gastric varices: expert review. *Clin Gastroenterol Hepatol*. 2021;19(6):1098-1107.

ALGORITHM 44.1 Management of patients with gastric varices *(GV)*. *BRTO*, Balloon-occluded retrograde transvenous obliteration; *GOV*, gastroesophageal varices; *HE*, hepatic encephalopathy; *IGV*, isolated gastric varices; *NSBB*, nonselective beta-blockers; *TIPS*, transjugular intrahepatic portosystemic shunt.

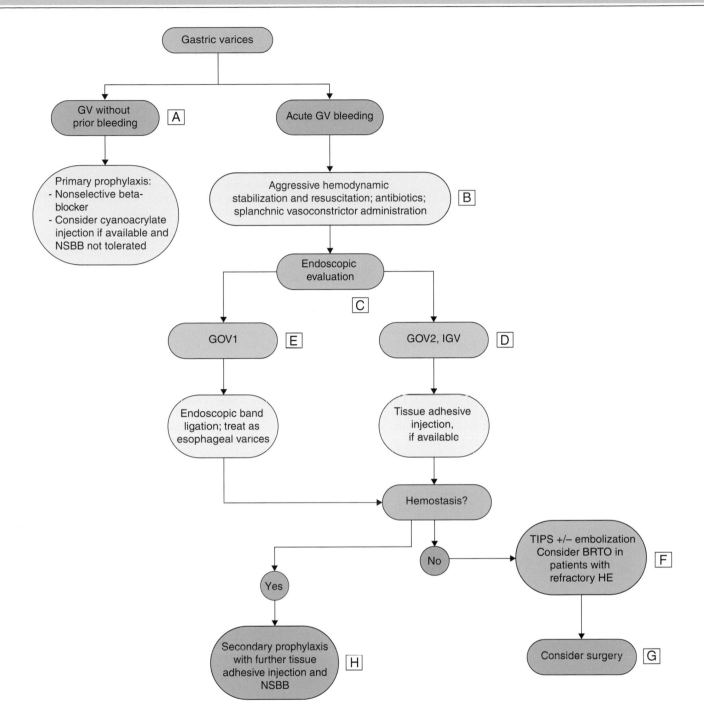

45 Chronic Bleeding From Portal Hypertension

Nikrad Shahnavaz

Portal hypertensive gastropathy (PHG) and gastric vascular ectasia (GVE) are the common causes of chronic gastrointestinal blood loss and iron deficiency anemia in patients with portal hypertension. These are two distinct mucosal lesions with different histologic features as well as different response to treatments.

A. PHG is recognized endoscopically by the presence of a mosaic-like pattern of the gastric mucosa (mild PHG), with or without superimposed discrete red and hemorrhagic spots or petechiae (severe PHG). PHG is mostly seen in the proximal stomach. Development of PHG correlates with the duration of cirrhosis rather than the degree of liver dysfunction.

B. In GVE, aggregates of ectatic vessels are seen during endoscopy, usually in the distal stomach (gastric antral vascular ectasia—GAVE) as red spots without a mosaic background. Watermelon stomach is the term used to describe GAVE when the lesions in the antrum are linear. If the endoscopic diagnosis is unclear, mucosal biopsies are recommended to differentiate GVE from gastritis. The biopsy in GVE demonstrates dilated mucosal capillaries with focal areas of fibrin thrombi in combination with proliferation of spindle cells. While about 30% of patients with GAVE have underlying cirrhosis, it has been associated with non-alcoholic fatty liver disease (without cirrhosis) as well as systemic sclerosis, chronic renal failure, acute myeloid leukemia, and cardiac diseases.

C. Primary prophylaxis is not recommended for asymptomatic patients with PHG, regardless of severity. Iron supplement and pharmacologic therapy with beta-blockers are recommended in patients with anemia who have bled from severe PHG.

D. If anemia persists and the patient requires frequent transfusions despite optimal drug therapy, a transjugular intrahepatic portosystemic shunt (TIPS) is recommended, which can result in reversal of the mucosal lesions and reduction of the blood transfusion requirement.

E. Bleeding from GVE is unrelated to portal hypertension; therefore, beta-blockers and TIPS are not helpful in controlling bleeding. The first line of treatment for patients with GVE and mild iron deficiency anemia is iron replacement. No further pharmacologic or endoscopic therapy is necessary if hemoglobin levels respond to iron supplement and occasional blood transfusion.

F. In patients with refractory anemia and localized GVE, thermoablative therapy with argon plasma coagulation (energy level of 60–90 W and a gas flow rate of 1–2 L/min) is recommended, if the platelet count is above 45,000/mm^3, and the international normalized ratio (INR) is less than 1.4. Endoscopic band ligation is emerging as a safe and effective treatment for GVE in patients with cirrhosis. Endoscopic therapy is performed every 2 weeks until complete obliteration of GVE is achieved.

G. When the coagulation parameters are suboptimal, the patient has extensive GVE involving the entire stomach, or endoscopic treatment does not control the chronic bleeding, an estrogen-progesterone therapy (e.g., estradiol 35 mcg plus norethindrone 1 mg daily) may be useful to reduce the requirement for blood transfusion.

H. GVE is reversed after liver transplantation, even in the presence of portal hypertension, suggesting that it is a consequence of liver failure, rather than portal hypertension. For this reason, TIPS has no role in the treatment of GVE.

I. In patients with refractory GAVE who are not a candidate for liver transplant, surgical antrectomy is rarely considered, although the postoperative risk of morbidity and mortality is significant in patients with severe liver disease. Also, some studies have shown the benefit of intravenous bevacizumab in reducing the requirement for blood transfusions, iron infusions, and endoscopic interventions in patients with refractory GAVE.

BIBLIOGRAPHY

1. Shah VH, Kamath PS Portal hypertension and variceal bleeding. Sleisenger and Fordtran's Gastrointestinal and Liver Disease. 11th Edition, Elsevier, 2020.
2. Kamath PS, Shah VH Portal hypertension related to bleeding. Zakim and Boyer's Hepatology. 7th Edition, Elsevier, 2016.
3. Abdo M., Moustafa A., Mostafa I., et al. To coagulate, ligate, or both: a randomized study comparing the safety and efficacy of two endoscopic approaches for managing gastric antral vascular ectasia in cirrhotic patients. *Egypt Liver Journal.* 2022;12:8. https://doi.org/10.1186/s43066-022-00173-4.
4. Elhendawy M, Mosaad S, Alkhalawany W, et al. Randomized controlled study of endoscopic band ligation and argon plasma coagulation in the treatment of gastric antral and fundal vascular ectasia. *United European Gastroenterol J.* 2016;4(3):423-428. https://doi.org/10.1177/2050640615619837.

ALGORITHM 45.1 Management of chronic bleeding from portal hypertension. *GAVE,* Gastric antral vascular ectasia; *GVE,* gastric vascular ectasia; *INR,* international normalized ratio; *PHG,* portal hypertensive gastropathy; *TIPS,* transjugular intrahepatic portosystemic shunt.

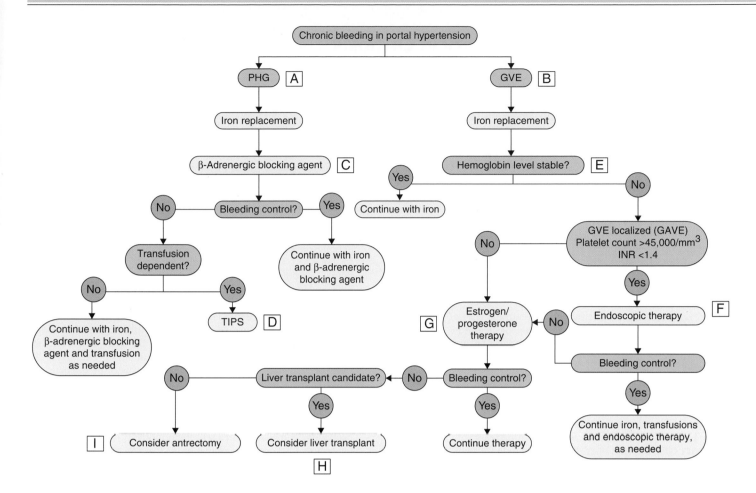

46 Acute Kidney Injury in Cirrhosis

Emad Qayed

Acute kidney injury (AKI) occurs in 15%–25% of patients hospitalized with cirrhosis. The main causes are prerenal azotemia (renal hypoperfusion) and acute tubular necrosis. Post-renal azotemia (urinary obstruction) is an uncommon cause of kidney injury in cirrhosis (<1%). Hepatorenal syndrome (HRS) accounts for 10%–30% of cases of AKI in cirrhosis and represents a distinct form of renal hypoperfusion that occurs in patients with cirrhosis and ascites with portal hypertension. In these patients, the circulatory dysfunction and splanchnic vasodilation lead to a state of perceived hypovolemia, which triggers the renin-angiotensin system. This leads to renal vasoconstriction, and decreased renal perfusion. This prerenal type of kidney injury does not respond to volume expansion. The same hemodynamic changes are responsible for the retention of sodium and water leading to the formation of ascites. HRS is now referred to as AKI-HRS.

A. AKI is defined as increase in serum creatinine (Cr) of ≥ 0.3 mg/dL within 48 hours; or a percentage increase of creatinine $\geq 50\%$ from baseline, which is presumed or known to have occurred within the past 7 days.

B. All patients should have a clinical assessment to evaluate for hypovolemia, and underlying infection (e.g., spontaneous bacterial peritonitis). Urine examination includes a routine urine analysis, electrolytes, and examination for urine sediment. Renal ultrasound is often used for evaluation, especially in patients with suspicion of urinary obstruction. Other measures include stopping any nephrotoxic drugs, diuretics, and lactulose, as appropriate.

C. If a specific diagnosis is made upon the initial evaluation (urinary tract infection or obstruction, acute tubular necrosis), then it should be treated accordingly.

D. If a specific diagnosis is not made and the AKI is mild (stage 1 AKI), it is appropriate to continue risk factor modifications and monitor for 1–2 days.

E. If a specific diagnosis is not made and the AKI is stage 2 or stage 3, diuretics should be stopped, and albumin should be administered for volume expansion for 48 hours.

F. If the AKI does not improve or resolve, most patients will fit the definition of HRS. The criteria for the diagnosis of HRS are: (1) cirrhosis with ascites, (2) diagnosis of AKI, (3) no response after 2 consecutive days of diuretic withdrawal and plasma volume expansion with albumin infusion, (4) absence of shock, (5) no current or recent use of nephrotoxic drugs, (6) no signs of structural kidney injury (absence of proteinuria, microhematuria, and/or abnormal renal ultrasound).

G. The management of HRS includes albumin infusion, and vasopressor therapy (terlipressin; midodrine and octreotide, or norepinephrine). Terlipressin is the preferred first line vasopressor agent for the treatment for HRS-AKI. It is given at a dose of 1 mg intravenously (IV) every 6 hours. Norepinephrine is given as a continuous IV infusion of 0.5 mg/hour, and the dose can be increased by 0.5 mg/hour every 4 hours up to 3 mg/hour. The drug should be titrated to achieve an increase in mean arterial pressure of >10 mm Hg. Midodrine and octreotide are inferior to terlipressin but can be used if terlipressin is unavailable. Midodrine is given at 2.5–5 mg orally every 8 hours, and the dose can be increased gradually up to 15 mg every 8 hours. Octreotide is given as 100–200 mcg subcutaneously every 8 hours. Patients should be evaluated for liver transplantation. Consider renal replacement therapy (RRT) in patients who do not respond to pharmacologic therapy and are on the liver transplant waiting list. RRT is considered as a bridge to transplantation, and its use is controversial in patients who are not candidates for transplantation, as it is associated with high mortality. All patients should be evaluated for liver transplantation, as this remains the treatment of choice for patients with AKI-HRS.

BIBLIOGRAPHY

1. Biggins SW, Angeli P, Garcia-Tsao G, et al. Diagnosis, evaluation, and management of ascites, spontaneous bacterial peritonitis and hepatorenal syndrome: 2021 practice guidance by the American Association for the Study of Liver Diseases. *Hepatology.* 2021;74(2):1014–1048.
2. Angeli P, Gines P, Wong F, et al. International Club of Ascites. Diagnosis and management of acute kidney injury in patients with cirrhosis: revised consensus recommendations of the International Club of Ascites. *Gut.* 2015;64(4):531–537.
3. Nadim MK, Garcia-Tsao G. Acute kidney injury in patients with cirrhosis. *N Engl J Med.* 2023;388(8):733–745. https://doi.org/10.1056/NEJMra2215289.

ALGORITHM 46.1 Flowchart for the workup and diagnosis of a patient with cirrhosis and acute kidney injury (AKI). *ACEI,* angiotensin-converting enzyme inhibitors; *ARB,* angiotensin receptor blockers; *CBC,* complete blood count; *Cr,* creatinine; *NSAIDs,* nonsteroidal antiinflammatory drugs; *US,* ultrasound.

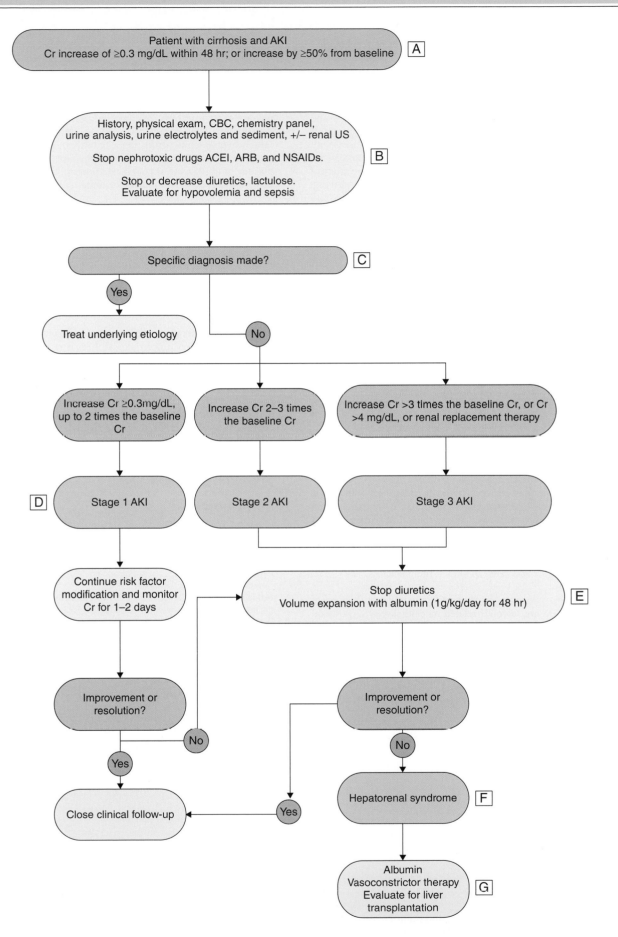

47 Hepatic Encephalopathy

Emad Qayed

Hepatic encephalopathy (HE) refers to the reversible neurologic and psychiatric manifestations that occur due to hepatic insufficiency and/or portal hypertension. Overt HE develops in 50%–70% of patients with cirrhosis, and it indicates a poor prognosis, with estimated 1- and 3-year survival rates of 42% and 23%, respectively. Patients develop a variety of symptoms that range from subtle (covert HE) such as difficulty driving, minor abnormalities of visual perception and psychometric testing, and sleep abnormalities, to more severe symptoms (overt HE) up to profound stupor and coma. The management of overt HE focuses on ruling out other etiologies of altered mental status, evaluation for precipitating factors, and specific therapy with lactulose and/or rifaximin.

A. The initial evaluation of a patient with cirrhosis and altered mental status should include a full history and physical examination. Neurologic examination should focus on cranial nerve examination and presence or absence of focal neurologic deficits. Clinical manifestations in overt HE include hyperreflexia, hypertonia, asterixis, rigidity, tremor, gait abnormalities, and seizures. Other manifestations include agitation, disorientation to time and place, slurred speech, lethargy, and apathy. Laboratory workup should include a complete blood count, full chemistry panels, and urine analysis. Blood cultures should be obtained if sepsis is suspected. In patients with ascites, paracentesis should be performed to rule out spontaneous bacterial peritonitis (SBP). In patients with known liver disease and suspected HE; measurement of serum ammonia level should be avoided because it does not change management or prognosis. In patients without known cirrhosis and portal hypertension, elevated serum ammonia level may indicate the presence of HE; however, nonhepatic hyperammonemia may occur in critically ill patients with sepsis, kidney disease, gastrointestinal bleeding, and in patients receiving valproic acid, carbamazepine, or corticosteroids. Brain imaging with computed tomography or magnetic resonance imaging should be considered if there are focal neurologic deficits and a suspicion of cerebrovascular events. Electroencephalogram (EEG) is useful to exclude postictal state as a cause of altered mental status.

B. If the initial workup leads to an alternative diagnosis such as acute cerebrovascular events, alcohol-related encephalopathy, postictal state, or metabolic encephalopathy (e.g., hypoglycemia, uremia), management should proceed to address these specific conditions.

C. In patients with confirmed overt HE, precipitating factors should be sought and treated to reverse HE. These include sepsis (SBP, urinary tract infection, pneumonia), gastrointestinal hemorrhage, constipation, dietary protein overload, dehydration, acute kidney injury, hypokalemia, drugs (e.g., sedatives), poor compliance with lactulose therapy, transjugular intrahepatic portosystemic shunt placement (TIPS), intestinal obstruction or ileus, portal vein thrombosis, and development of hepatocellular carcinoma.

D. Patients with HE who can protect their airway are usually admitted to the general floor. Oral lactulose is administered, and rectal lactulose is an alternative if the patient cannot tolerate oral administration.

E. Patients with advanced HE who are not able to protect their airway should be admitted to the intensive care unit, and endotracheal intubation should be performed. Lactulose can be administered through a nasogastric or orogastric tube.

F. Patients who improve on lactulose should be given maintenance lactulose for secondary prophylaxis. If there is recurrent HE (>2 previous HE episodes), then rifaximin should be added to lactulose as a maintenance therapy to decrease the incidence of recurrence.

G. In patients who do not improve on lactulose, rifaximin should be added to the treatment regimen. If lactulose is not tolerated, it should be discontinued and rifaximin continued as monotherapy. The diagnosis of HE should be confirmed by reevaluating the workup for a missed alternative diagnosis or precipitating factor. Other treatments of HE with less clear benefit include zinc, L-ornithine-L-aspartate, polyethylene glycol, and acarbose.

BIBLIOGRAPHY

1. Handbook of Liver Disease, Fourth Edition, Copyright © 2018 by Elsevier; Chapter 15: Hepatic encephalopathy.
2. Sleisenger and Fordtran's Gastrointestinal and Liver Disease, Eleventh Edition, Copyright © 2021 by Elsevier. Chapter 94: Hepatic Encephalopathy, Hepatorenal Syndrome, Hepatopulmonary Syndrome, and Other Systemic Complications of Liver Disease.
3. Patidar KR, Bajaj JS. Covert and overt hepatic encephalopathy: diagnosis and management. *Clin Gastroenterol Hepatol.* 2015;13(12):2048-2061.
4. Haj M, Rockey DC. Ammonia levels do not guide clinical management of patients with hepatic encephalopathy caused by cirrhosis. *Am J Gastroenterol.* 2020;115:723.
5. Zhao L, Walline JH, Gao Y, et al. Prognostic role of ammonia in critical care patients without known hepatic disease. *Front Med (Lausanne).* 2020;7:589825.

ALGORITHM 47.1 Flowchart for the workup and diagnosis of a patient with cirrhosis and altered mental status jaundice. *BM*, Bowel movement; *CBC*, complete blood count; *HE*, hepatic encephalopathy.

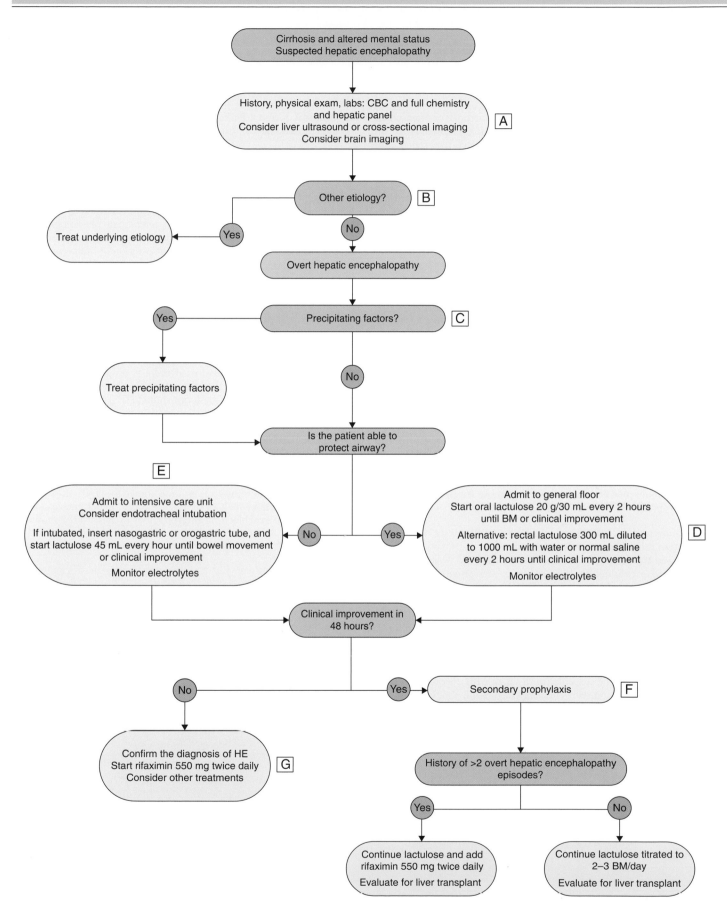

48 Portal Vein Thrombosis in Cirrhosis

Michael Andrew Yu

Portal vein thrombosis (PVT) in patients with cirrhosis is often noted incidentally during hepatocellular carcinoma (HCC) screening. It can contribute to the development or worsening of portal hypertension in these patients.

A. After identification, a detailed history and physical examination should be obtained to assess for any evidence of decompensated cirrhosis, any history of thrombophilia or HCC. The severity of cirrhosis should be noted as should any prior endoscopic sclerotherapy of esophageal varices. Prior imaging should be reviewed to assess chronicity of the thrombus. Next, further cross-sectional imaging with a contrasted computed tomography (CT) or magnetic resonance imaging (MRI) should be obtained.

B. If there is presence of HCC, tumoral involvement of the portal vein must be assessed. The A-VENA criteria can help diagnose a tumoral PVT and distinguish it from a nontumoral PVT. The criteria include the following: Alpha fetoprotein (AFP) >1000, Venous expansions, thrombus Enhancement, Neovascularity, and Adjacency to HCC. The presence of ≥3 criteria distinguish tumoral PVT with high accuracy and the patient should be evaluated by interventional radiology and oncology for locoregional or systemic therapy.

C. The portal vein thrombus should be described temporally (acute or chronic), by extent (percent occlusion of main portal vein, and involvement of other mesenteric veins), and if noted previously, by interval change (progression, stable, or regression). Typically, an acute PVT is <6 months, while chronic one is >6 months in duration. The presence of cavernoma or cavernous transformation indicates a chronic PVT.

D. There are several classification systems for PVT and the Yerdel classification is one that is commonly used.
   a. Grade 1: Minimal or partially thrombosed PV where thrombus is mild or confined to <50% of lumen with or without extension into superior mesenteric vein (SMV)
   b. Grade 2: >50% occlusion including total occlusion with or without minimal extension into SMV
   c. Grade 3: Complete thrombosis of both PV and proximal SMV
   d. Grade 4: Complete thrombosis of PV and both proximal and distal SMV

E. Grade 1 PVTs can be surveilled with CT or MRI every 3 months to assess for progression. However, anticoagulation should be initiated if the patient is awaiting liver transplant or if there is thrombus involvement of the SMV.

F. Grades 2, 3, and 4 PVTs, or progressive PVTs should be started on anticoagulation.

G. Low-molecular-weight heparin is the treatment of choice, but vitamin K antagonists can be used. Direct oral anticoagulants (DOACs) can be used except in patients with Child-Pugh C cirrhosis.

H. If there is complete obstruction of PV with extension into the SMV, and the patient receives an organ offer, then physiological portal-to-portal vein anastomosis during transplant is prevented. Alternatives include a portocaval hemitransposition or a left renal vein to graft portal vein anastomosis.

I. The PVT should be reevaluated in 3-6 months while on anticoagulation. If there is improvement, the anticoagulation can be continued. There is no current standard for duration of anticoagulation as recurrence of thrombosis can occur in complete recanalization after 2-5 months following discontinuing anticoagulation.

J. If there is no improvement or if there is progression of the PVT despite anticoagulation, then the patient should be referred for transjugular intrahepatic portosystemic shunt (TIPS) and possible thrombolysis. TIPS can achieve partial and complete resolution of a PVT with a success rate of 75%-98%. In the presence of an extensive PVT, a mechanical thrombolysis during the TIPS can be considered. TIPS can also be considered if there is any contraindication to anticoagulation.

K. If the patient develops other indications for TIPS at any time during evaluation, such as significant portal hypertensive complications as variceal bleeding and refractory ascites, a TIPS should be considered.

BIBLIOGRAPHY

1. European Association for the Study of the Liver EASL clinical practice guidelines: vascular diseases of the liver. *J Hepatol.* 2016;64(1):179–202.
2. Northup PG, Garcia-Pagan JC, Garcia-Tsao G, et al. Vascular liver disorders, portal vein thrombosis, and procedural bleeding in patients with liver disease: 2020 Practice Guidance by the American Association for the Study of Liver Diseases. *Hepatology.* 2021;73(1):366–413.
3. Sarin SK, Philips CA, Kamath PS, et al. Toward a comprehensive new classification of portal vein thrombosis in patients with cirrhosis. *Gastroenterology.* 2016;151(4):574–577.e3.
4. Senzolo M, Garcia-Tsao G, García-Pagán JC. Current knowledge and management of portal vein thrombosis in cirrhosis. *J Hepatol.* 2021;75(2):442–453.

ALGORITHM 48.1 Management of portal vein thrombosis in cirrhosis. *CT,* Computed tomography; *DOAC,* direct oral anticoagulant; *HCC,* hepatocellular carcinoma; *LT,* liver transplantation; *MRI,* magnetic resonance imaging; *SMV,* superior mesenteric vein; *TIPS,* transjugular intrahepatic portosystemic shunt; *PVT,* portal vein thrombosis.

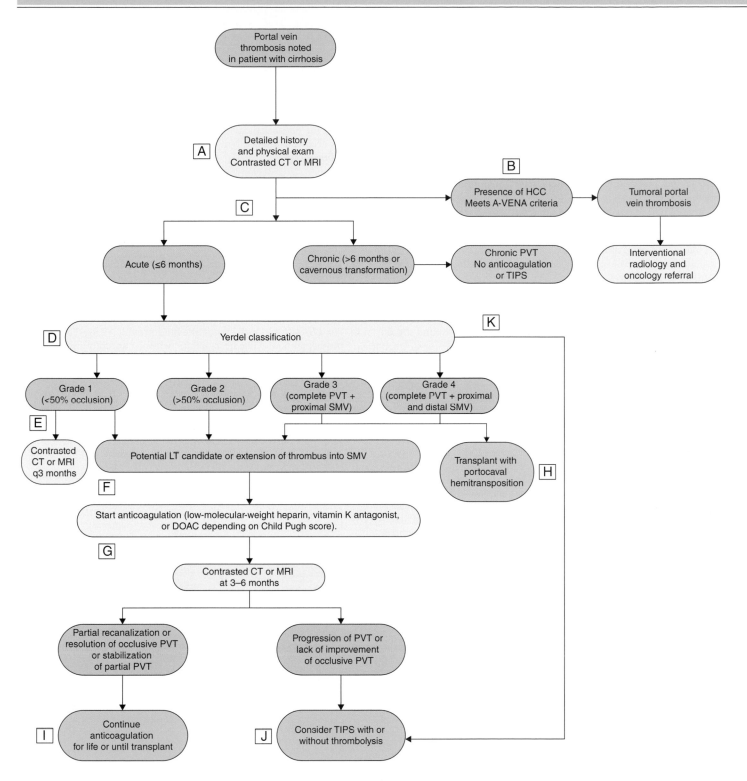

Ascites

Michael Andrew Yu

Ascites, or the accumulation of fluid within the peritoneal cavity, is most commonly caused by cirrhosis, which accounts for about 80% of cases. It occurs as a complication of portal hypertension, which drives splanchnic vasodilation leading to a reduced effective arterial circulation, renal sodium retention, and volume overload. Other causes of ascites include heart failure, pancreatic disease, malignancy, nephrotic syndrome, and tuberculous peritonitis.

A. Initial history should focus on questions about liver disease, heart failure, pancreatitis, cancer, travel to countries endemic for tuberculosis, and renal disease. The physical examination of the abdomen should include evaluation for flank or shifting dullness and inspecting for signs of cirrhosis such as palmar erythema, spider telangiectasias, or jaundice. Also critical are auscultating the heart and lungs, palpating for any abdominal masses, and checking for jugular venous distention and presence of peripheral edema. Laboratory assessment of renal and hepatic function, and an abdominal ultrasound should be pursued.

B. A diagnostic paracentesis is critical in evaluating the cause of ascites. The appearance of the ascites fluid should be noted (clear, bloody, or milky—suggestive of chylous ascites). Ascitic fluid should be sent for cell count with differential, total protein and albumin concentration, and culture. A polymorphonuclear neutrophil count of ≥ 250 cells/mm^3 is diagnostic for spontaneous bacterial peritonitis and warrants antibiotics (refer to Chapter 50—Spontaneous Bacterial Peritonitis). A fluid culture should be obtained by inoculating ≥ 10 mL of fluid into blood culture bottles immediately after paracentesis. Other tests of ascitic fluid such as triglycerides, and amylase levels can be performed selectively if chylous ascites or pancreatic ascites is suspected, respectively. Mycobacterial culture should be performed if tuberculosis is suspected. Ascitic fluid cytology can aid in the diagnosis when malignancy is suspected as the cause of ascites. Chylous ascites is described as the ascitic fluid that has a milky appearance, with a high triglyceride level (>200 mg/dL). It is caused by the rupture of intra-abdominal lymphatic vessels and leakage of lipid-rich lymph into the peritoneal cavity. Possible etiologies include cirrhosis, retroperitoneal surgery, lymphoma, intra-abdominal malignancy, and tuberculosis.

C. The serum-ascites albumin gradient (SAAG) is calculated by subtracting the ascitic fluid albumin level from the serum albumin level; and a value ≥ 1.1 g/dL indicates a portal hypertension-related ascites (e.g., cirrhosis), while a value <1.1 g/dL indicates a nonportal hypertension-related etiology.

D. The ascitic protein concentration can help further narrow down the etiology of ascites. For a SAAG <1.1 g/dL, an ascitic fluid protein ≥ 2.5 g/dL could be from malignancy or tuberculosis, while a concentration <2.5 g/dL suggests nephrotic syndrome.

E. For a SAAG ≥ 1.1 g/dL, an ascitic fluid protein ≥ 2.5 g/dL suggests a posthepatic cause like heart failure, while a concentration <2.5 g/dL suggests a sinusoidal cause like cirrhosis or prehepatic cause like a portal vein thrombosis.

BIBLIOGRAPHY

1. Biggins SW, Angeli P, Garcia-Tsao G, et al. Diagnosis, evaluation, and management of ascites, spontaneous bacterial peritonitis and hepatorenal syndrome: 2021 practice guidance by the American Association for the Study of Liver Diseases. *Hepatology.* 2021;74(2):1014-1048.
2. European Association for the Study of the Liver EASL Clinical Practice Guidelines for the management of patients with decompensated cirrhosis. *J Hepatol.* 2018;69(2):406-460. Erratum in: J Hepatol. 2018;69(5):1207.
3. Sleisenger and Fordtran's Gastrointestinal and Liver Disease, Eleventh Edition, Elsevier, 2021. Chapter 93: Ascites and Spontaneous Bacterial Peritonitis
4. Bhardwaj R, Vaziri H, Gautam A, Ballesteros E, Karimeddini D, Wu GY. Chylous ascites: a review of pathogenesis, diagnosis and treatment. *J Clin Transl Hepatol.* 2018;6(1):105-113. https://doi.org/10.14218/JCTH.2017.00035.

ALGORITHM 49.1 Flowchart for the workup and diagnosis of a patient with ascites. *AFB,* Acid-fast bacilli; *CBC,* complete blood count; *CMP,* comprehensive metabolic panel; *CT,* computed tomography; *MRI,* magnetic resonance imaging; *SAAG,* serum-ascites albumin gradient; *US,* ultrasound.

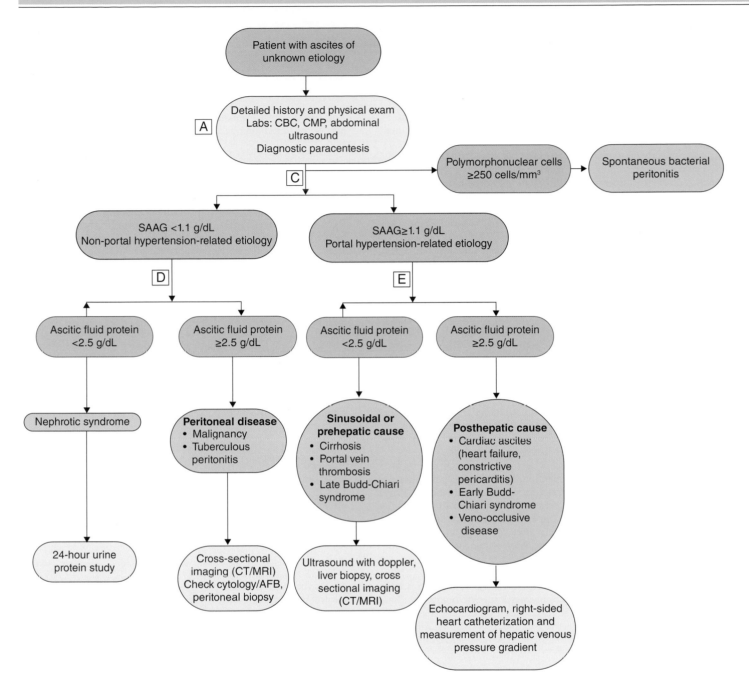

50 Spontaneous Bacterial Peritonitis

Emad Qayed

Spontaneous bacterial peritonitis (SBP) is defined as bacterial infection of the ascitic fluid without any specific identifiable intraabdominal source of infection. The prognosis of SBP has improved over the years as a result of early diagnosis and appropriate management. Patients with SBP can develop abdominal pain, vomiting, diarrhea, or can be asymptomatic. They can also present with signs of systemic inflammation, deterioration of liver function, hepatic encephalopathy, acute kidney injury (AKI), or septic shock. A diagnostic paracentesis should be performed to evaluate for SBP in all patients with cirrhosis and ascites who are admitted to the hospital, and in those who develop complications such as gastrointestinal bleeding, hepatic encephalopathy, and AKI. The optimal management of SBP requires early diagnosis and antibiotic treatment to improve outcomes.

A. The diagnosis of SBP is based on the neutrophil count in ascitic fluid of >250/mm^3. A positive culture is not necessary for the diagnosis of SBP; however, it can guide the proper antibiotic treatment. If bacterial fluid culture is positive with monomicrobial growth, and neutrophil count in ascitic fluid is <250/mm^3, this condition is also treated as SBP. The choice of empiric antibiotic treatment depends on the setting in which the infection is acquired and the severity of illness.

B. In patients with mild community-acquired infection, without recent exposure to antibiotics, third-generation cephalosporins (cefotaxime or ceftriaxone) are appropriate. If there is severe infection (e.g., sepsis), then piperacillin-tazobactam is used for treatment.

C. In patients with nosocomial infection, or with severe healthcare-acquired infection with sepsis, meropenem is recommended. Vancomycin can be added to the treatment regimen if there is high prevalence of methicillin-resistant *Staphylococcus aureus* (MRSA) and vancomycin-susceptible enterococci. Daptomycin or linezolid is added in areas with a high prevalence of vancomycin-resistant enterococci.

D. Albumin therapy at 1.5 g/kg IV on day 1, and 1 g/kg on day 3 is recommended in SBP. If fluid culture grows a specific organism, then antibiotic therapy should be adjusted based on culture results and overall clinical status. Nonselective beta blockers (NSBBs) should be temporarily held in patients with SBP who develop AKI or hypoten-

sion (mean arterial pressure <65 mm Hg). If discontinued, NSBBs may be restarted after recovery of the kidney injury and hypotension.

E. If there is clinical improvement within 48 hours, then antibiotics should be continued for 5 days and then discontinued.

F. If there is no clinical improvement in 48 hours (e.g., persistent pain, fever, deteriorating clinical status), then repeat paracentesis should be performed to evaluate treatment response. If neutrophil count in ascitic fluid is <250/mm^3, then antibiotics should be continued for 5 days, and alternate sources of infection should be sought.

G. If repeat paracentesis reveals neutrophil count >250/mm^3, then antibiotics should be adjusted and usually coverage is broadened to cover multidrug-resistant organisms.

H. Secondary prophylaxis is indicated in patients with a history of SBP. Antibiotic regimens include norfloxacin, trimethoprim-sulfamethoxazole, and ciprofloxacin. Ascites should be treated with diuretics. Proton pump inhibitor use has been associated with SBP in cirrhosis, and they should be restricted to patients with strong indications for their use. Patients should be referred for liver transplant evaluation.

BIBLIOGRAPHY

1. Sleisenger and Fordtran's Gastrointestinal and Liver Disease, Eleventh Edition, Elsevier, 2021. Chapter 93 – Ascites and Spontaneous Bacterial Peritonitis.
2. European Association for the Study of the Liver EASL Clinical Practice Guidelines for the management of patients with decompensated cirrhosis. *J Hepatol*. 2018;69(2):406-460. Erratum in: J Hepatol. 2018;69(5):1207.
3. Dever JB, Sheikh MY. Review article: spontaneous bacterial peritonitis–bacteriology, diagnosis, treatment, risk factors and prevention. *Aliment Pharmacol Ther*. 2015;41(11):1116-1131.
4. Biggins SW, Angeli P, Garcia-Tsao G, et al. Diagnosis, evaluation, and management of ascites, spontaneous bacterial peritonitis and hepatorenal syndrome: 2021 practice guidance by the American Association for the Study of Liver Diseases. *Hepatology*. 2021;74(2):1014-1048.

ALGORITHM 50.1 Flowchart for empirical antibiotic treatment in spontaneous bacterial peritonitis *(SBP)*. *IV*, Intravenous; *PMN*: polymorphonuclear neutrophils; *PPI*: proton pump inhibitors.

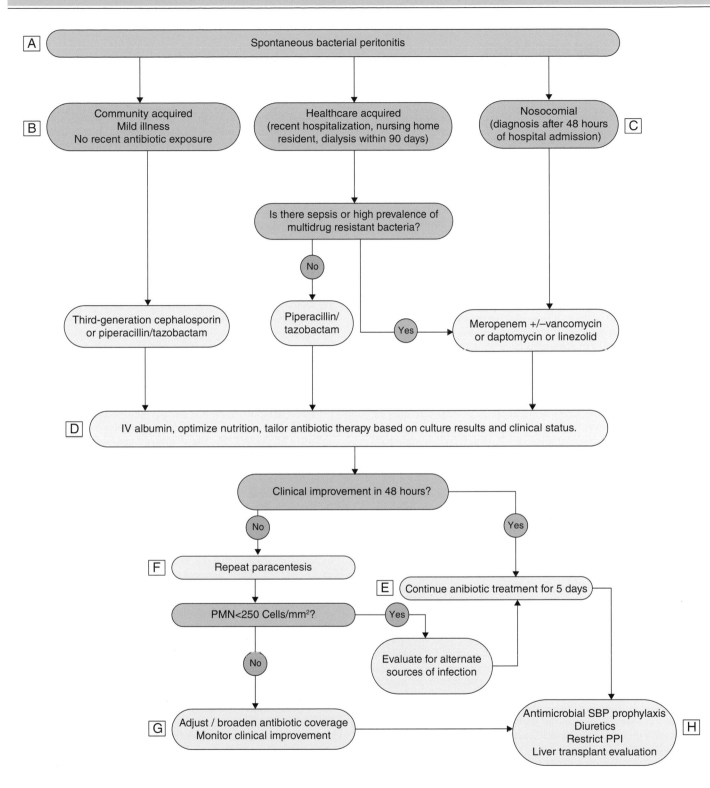

51 Hepatic Mass

Giorgio Roccaro

Hepatic lesions are commonly detected on imaging studies performed for an unrelated reason. Lesions can vary from solid to cystic and include benign and malignant entities. The diagnostic approach is centered on whether the detected mass is solid or cystic and whether the patient has a history of risk factors for hepatic malignancy. Diagnostic imaging of solid liver lesions generally begins with contrast-enhanced, multiphasic cross-sectional modalities such as computed tomography (CT) or magnetic resonance imaging (MRI).

A. Cystic lesions are rarely malignant. The most common is the simple liver cyst, a cystic formation containing clear fluid that does not communicate with the biliary tree. Ultrasonography and/or cross-sectional imaging with CT or MRI can distinguish a simple cyst from other cystic liver lesions. For asymptomatic patients with simple liver cysts, no intervention or surveillance is required as these lesions do not have malignant potential irrespective of size. Patients with large, symptomatic liver cysts may require intervention if all other potential causes of symptoms have been excluded. Simple liver cysts are most likely to be symptomatic when large (≥4 cm) and located in the left hepatic lobe adjacent to the stomach and proximal to the small intestine. In this scenario, mass effect on the upper digestive track can lead to symptoms of early satiety, abdominal distention, and weight loss. Cross-sectional contrast-enhanced imaging with CT or MRI is most commonly used to distinguish other forms of hepatic cystic lesions (complex cysts), which include mucinous cystic neoplasm (MCN), echinococcal cyst, ciliated hepatic foregut cyst, and biliary cysts.

B. For a patient with an incidental solid liver mass, it is critical to determine if the patient is at increased risk for hepatocellular carcinoma (HCC) or liver metastases. Patients with chronic advanced liver disease marked by advanced hepatic fibrosis or cirrhosis as well as those with chronic hepatitis B infection are at increased risk for HCC. Those with a history of extrahepatic malignancy, particularly of advanced stage, are at increased risk for liver metastases. The evaluation of these patients differs from those without these corresponding risk factors.

C. Cross-sectional contrast-enhanced imaging, either by MRI or CT, is often necessary to characterize solid liver lesions. Most liver lesions have characteristic enhancement features, which can distinguish the etiology without invasive testing. The most common benign solid liver masses occurring in patients without risk factors for hepatic malignancy include hepatic hemangioma, hepatocellular adenoma (HCA), and focal nodular hyperplasia (FNH). Histologic evaluation via percutaneous biopsy can be performed if imaging is unable to definitively make a diagnosis or to exclude malignant transformation of an adenoma.

D. Hepatic hemangioma is the most common benign liver lesion. They occur more frequently in women. Hemangiomas are rarely symptomatic or warranting of intervention. It can be diagnosed with noncontrast ultrasound or contrast-enhanced CT or MRI. On MRI, hemangiomas appear as a well-demarcated homogeneous mass with low signal intensity of T1 weighted images and T2 hyperintensity. With contrast, they enhance peripherally in the arterial phase. On contrast-enhanced CT, hemangiomas demonstrate peripheral nodular enhancement in the early phase followed by a progressive filling

in during the late phase. Finally, they remain hyperdense in delayed phases. A hemangioma is classified as "giant" if it is greater than 10 cm. Lesions less than 5 cm require no further surveillance. Lesions greater than 5 cm are more likely to cause symptoms if they are growing rapidly (i.e., growth rate >3 mm/year). Surveillance imaging at an interval of 6–12 months is recommended to monitor hemangiomas over 5 cm in size. Symptomatic patients may exhibit abdominal pain or early satiety due to mass effect. It is crucial to rule out other causes of these symptoms such as peptic ulcer disease, cholelithiasis, irritable bowel syndrome, or malignancy. Patients with symptoms or rapidly growing large hemangiomas should be evaluated by a hepatobiliary surgeon for consideration of surgical intervention.

E. FNH is a benign solid liver lesion composed of a proliferation of hyperplastic hepatocytes surrounding a central stellate scar. With a prevalence of 0.3%–3.0%, it is commonly discovered on abdominal cross-sectional imaging performed for other reasons. FNH is a benign entity, which requires no further surveillance. However, it can be difficult to distinguish from hepatic adenomas, which often do require surveillance. MRI with administration of a liver-specific gadolinium-based contrast agent can distinguish FNH from malignant and premalignant entities; FNH has a rapid enhancement due to its arterial blood supply and subsequently become more isointense with respect to normal liver on delayed sequences. The central scar enhances on delayed imaging as contrast gradually diffuses into the fibrous center of the mass.

F. HCA is a solid benign liver mass that develops in otherwise normal-appearing liver parenchyma. They are typically solitary and are found predominantly in women. They are associated with use of estrogen-containing medications such as oral contraception. Typically, HCAs are discovered as incidental imaging findings in asymptomatic individuals. However, they can be discovered during evaluation of episodic abdominal pain that may be localized to the epigastrium or right upper quadrant. Rarely, a patient may present with acute, life-threatening intraperitoneal hemorrhage due to HCA rupture. HCAs are usually well-demarcated masses on contrast-enhanced imaging because of fat or glycogen content of the hepatocytes. On MRI, they demonstrate arterial phase enhancement with subsequent centripetal flow during the portal venous phase. They may have areas of hemorrhage, necrosis, or fibrosis, giving them a heterogeneous appearance. Core needle biopsy is usually not indicated because HCA may be difficult to distinguish microscopically from normal hepatocytes. However, if there is concern for malignancy due to imaging characteristics (i.e., portal venous washout or pseudocapsule), a biopsy can be performed if there is no other indication for surgical resection. For all patients with HCA, discontinuation of estrogen-containing medications is recommended as this may result in lesion size regression. Asymptomatic women with lesions less than 5 cm are observed with surveillance cross-sectional imaging every 6–12 months. In women with symptomatic HCA or HCA >5 cm as well as men with any size HCA, surgical resection is typically recommended due to the greater risk of rupture or malignant transformation.

G. For patients at increased risk of HCC including those with cirrhosis, advanced hepatic fibrosis (F3), and chronic hepatitis B, imaging surveillance with ultrasound every 6 months is recommended in conjunction with alpha-fetoprotein (AFP) testing. For patients in whom ultrasound is limited by body habitus, hepatic steatosis, or severe

ALGORITHM 51.1 Approach to the hepatic mass. *CT*, Computed tomography; *FNH*, focal nodular hyperplasia; *LI-RADS*, Liver Imaging Reporting and Data System; *MRI*, magnetic resonance imaging; *PET*, positron emission tomography.

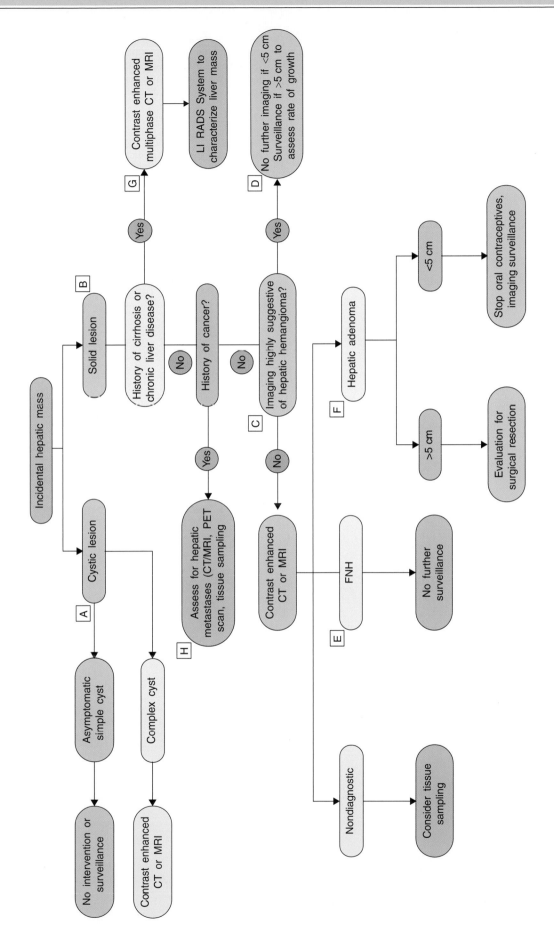

parenchymal heterogeneity from advanced cirrhosis, CT or MRI can be used as an alternative surveillance modality. Solid lesions >1 cm detected on ultrasound should be further evaluated with contrast-enhanced multiphasic cross-sectional imaging. HCC can be diagnosed on the basis of imaging alone in patients with morphologic changes or chronic liver disease as they may demonstrate characteristic findings of nonrim arterial phase hyperenhancement, nonperipheral washout in portal venous phase, and an enhancing capsule in the portal venous or delayed phase. The Liver Imaging Reporting and Data System (LI-RADS) is a system used for standardizing the characterization of liver lesions in patients with chronic liver disease. Refer to Chapter 52, Liver Lesions in Cirrhosis, for further discussion on diagnosis and management of these patients.

H. The liver is a common site for metastasis from solid tumors. Patients with a history of prior malignancy are at higher risk for hepatic metastasis. The enhancement pattern of liver metastases varies depending on the type of primary cancer. The presence of lesions in multiple organs or progression of cancer in the site of origin supports a diagnosis of metastatic disease. Image-guided liver biopsy is often useful to confirm the diagnosis.

BIBLIOGRAPHY

1. Marrero JA, Ahn J, Rajender Reddy K. American College of Gastroenterology. ACG clinical guideline: the diagnosis and management of focal liver lesions. *Am J Gastroenterol.* 2014;109(9):1328-1347.
2. Di Bisceglie AM, Befeler AS Hepatic tumors and cysts. Sleisenger and Fordtran's Gastrointestinal and Liver Disease. 11th Edition, Elsevier, 2020.
3. Zhang W, Di Bisceglie AM Hepatic tumors. Handbook of Liver Disease. 4th Edition, Elsevier, 2017.
4. Colombo M, Sangiovanni A, Lencioni R Benign liver tumors. Zakim and Boyer's Hepatology. 7th Edition, Elsevier, 2016.

52 | Liver Lesions in Cirrhosis

Emad Qayed

Screening for hepatocellular carcinoma (HCC) is recommended for patients with cirrhosis, and in some hepatitis B carriers (Asian males above the age of 40 years, Asian females above the age of 50 years, family history of HCC, and Africans/African Americans). A liver ultrasound with or without alpha-fetoprotein (AFP) every 6 months is recommended by the American Association for the Study of Liver Diseases (AASLD). In patients with obesity and/or inadequate ultrasound exam, it is reasonable to perform cross-sectional imaging for HCC screening. The AASLD does not recommend screening for HCC in patients with advanced cirrhosis (Child's class C) unless these patients are on the liver transplant list.

A. If a lesion is detected during routine ultrasound screening for HCC, further management depends on the size of the lesion. Of note, if AFP is elevated to a level >20 ng/mL, then cross-sectional imaging should be performed to examine for underlying lesions.

B. If the lesion is <1 cm in size, it is reasonable to repeat ultrasound in 3–6 months.

C. If the lesion is ≥1 cm in size, further workup with triphasic computed tomography (CT) or magnetic resonance imaging (MRI) is required.

D. Images must be interpreted through a structured system called the *Liver Imaging Reporting and Data System* (*LI-RADS*). The goal of this system is to standardize the reporting of all liver lesions in cirrhotic patients. The system categorizes each liver lesion according to its likelihood of malignancy, based on features of the lesions (diameter, arterial phase hyperenhancement, washout appearance, late hyperenhancement, capsule appearance, and threshold growth from prior imaging). Further management is based on the LI-RADS category (LR 1–5, LR-M, LR-NC). LR 2–4, LR-NC lesions require repeat imaging, which could be performed using the same or different modality (CT or MRI).

E. If the lesion is definitely benign, return to routine ultrasound screening every 6 months.

F. The risk of underlying malignancy increases as the LI-RADS category progresses from LR-2 to LR-4. However, it is unclear if the management of LR-2 should differ from LR-3 or LR-4. If the patient has a nodule and would be considered for HCC treatment if diagnosed, some experts recommend a diagnostic workup of these nodules, including biopsy.

G. For a lesion to be categorized as HCC, it has to fulfill certain imaging characteristics. For lesions that are ≥20 mm in size, the lesion is considered LI-RADS-5 if there is arterial phase hyperenhancement plus one or more of the following characteristics: (1) nonperipheral washout, (2) enhancing capsule appearance, and (3) threshold growth (defined as size increase by ≥50% in ≤6 months). For lesions that are 10–19 mm in size, the lesion is considered LI-RADS-5 if there is arterial phase hyperenhancement and all of the previous characteristics. LI-RADS-5 is considered definite HCC, and management should proceed accordingly, without the need for biopsy (see Chapter 53). In patients without cirrhosis, the diagnosis of HCC cannot be made by the presence of characteristic imaging features alone, and a biopsy is required for diagnosis.

H. If the lesion appears probably or definitely malignant, but not definitely HCC, it is classified as LI-RADS-M. These lesions require further workup based on multidisciplinary discussion, which may include biopsy or repeat imaging in ≤3 months.

BIBLIOGRAPHY

1. Zakim and Boyer's Hepatology, 7th Edition, Elsevier, 2018. Chapter 46, Hepatocellular carcinoma.
2. Marrero JA, Kulik LM, Sirlin CB, et al. Diagnosis, staging, and management of hepatocellular carcinoma: 2018 practice guidance by the American Association for the Study of Liver Diseases. *Hepatology*. 2018;68(2):723-750.
3. Bruix J, Ayuso C. Diagnosis of hepatic nodules in patients at risk for hepatocellular carcinoma: LI-RADS probability versus certainty. *Gastroenterology*. 2019;156(4):860-862.

ALGORITHM 52.1 Flowchart for the workup of liver lesions detected during ultrasound screening for hepatocellular carcinoma *(HCC)*. *CT*: Computed tomography; *LI-RADS*: Liver Imaging Reporting and Data System; *MRI*: magnetic resonance imaging.

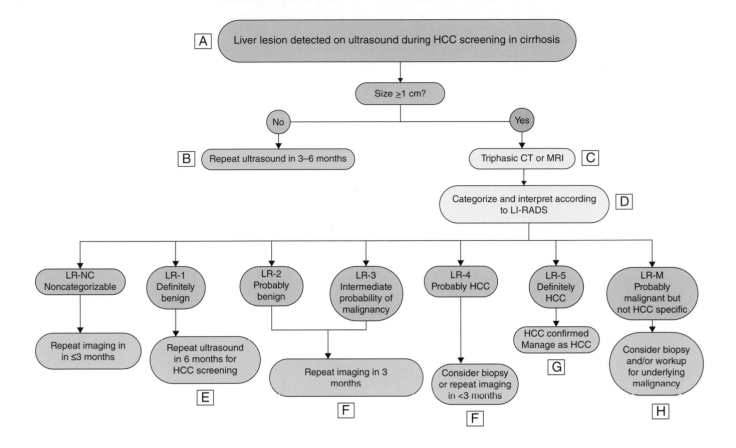

53 Hepatocellular Carcinoma

Emad Qayed

The suggested management of patients with hepatocellular carcinoma (HCC) is based on the stage of the tumor and degree of liver dysfunction. Staging is based on tumor size and spread, the patient's performance status (PS) as assessed by the Eastern Cooperative Oncology Group (ECOG) scale from 0 (good) to greater than 2 (poor), and liver function. Assessment of liver function is traditionally performed using the Child-Pugh score, in which patients with Child-Pugh class A and B are considered to have preserved liver function, while a patient with Child-Pugh class C is considered to have advanced liver disease. Other scores that are used to evaluate severity of liver disease are the albumin-bilirubin (ALBI) and the Model for End-Stage Liver Disease (MELD) score. All patients should be discussed in a multidisciplinary tumor board. The Barcelona Clinic Liver Cancer (BCLC) staging classification and treatment approach is commonly used for HCC.

A. Patients with very early (stage 0) HCC who are not potential candidates for liver transplant (LT) are ideal candidates for surgical resection if the bilirubin is normal and portal hypertension is absent. Large resections of the liver are possible if cirrhosis is absent. Only small resections (segmentectomy or enucleation) may be possible in a cirrhotic liver.

B. Patients with early (stage A) HCC are candidates for radical therapy. Options include resection, deceased-donor LT, or live-donor LT, or local ablation via percutaneous ethanol injection, radiofrequency ablation, or microwave ablation. LT is considered in patients who have an unresectable tumor that is confined to the liver, or if the tumor is resectable but patients are poor surgical candidates due to advanced cirrhosis with poor liver function. The Milan criteria are used to select patients for LT: one lesion <5 cm or up to three lesions each ≤3 cm, with no extrahepatic spread or vascular invasion. The 5-year survival rate in patients within Milan criteria who receive LT is 70%–75%, and the tumor recurrence rate is 10%–15%.

C. Patients with intermediate (stage B) HCC are candidates for transarterial chemoembolization (TACE). In this technique, chemotherapeutic agents are injected into the hepatic artery, which is subsequently occluded, which leads to shrinking of the tumor. TACE is used for patients with intermediate-stage HCC and preserved liver function, and can lead to downstaging the tumor to fit within the Milan criteria for liver transplantation. The BCLC has recently added a stratification for patients with HCC stage B. Patients who meet expanded liver transplant criteria are considered for LT, while those with more extensive disease involving both lobes of the liver are considered for systemic therapy instead of TACE.

D. Patients with advanced HCC stage C have presence of macroscopic vascular invasion, extrahepatic spread, or cancer-related symptoms, with ECOG PS 1 or 2. These patients are candidates for several systemic therapy options such as atezolizumab plus bevacizumab, sorafenib, lenvatinib, and nivolumab.

E. Patients with end-stage disease (stage D) should receive palliative care and symptomatic treatment.

BIBLIOGRAPHY

1. Handbook of Liver Disease, 4th Edition, Elsevier, 2018. Chapter 26, Hepatic tumors.
2. Sleisenger and Fordtran's Gastrointestinal and Liver Disease, 11th Edition, Elsevier, 2021. Chapter 96, Hepatic Tumors and Cysts.
3. Reig M, Forner A, Rimola J, et al. BCLC strategy for prognosis prediction and treatment recommendation: the 2022 update. *J Hepatol.* 2022;76(3):681-693.

ALGORITHM 53.1 Barcelona Clinic Liver Cancer (BCLC) staging classification and treatment approach for hepatocellular carcinoma. *ECOG,* Eastern Cooperative Oncology Group; *LT,* liver transplant; *PS,* performance status.

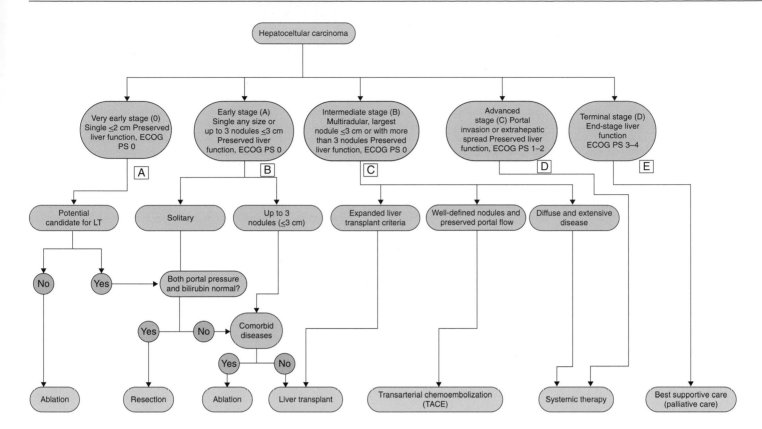

Suspected Choledocholithiasis

Emad Qayed

Patients with symptomatic gallstone disease present with episodic biliary pain, cholecystitis, or acute gallstone pancreatitis, and they are often suspected to have coexisting choledocholithiasis. The definitive treatment of gallstone disease is cholecystectomy.

A. The decision to further investigate the presence of choledocholithiasis before cholecystectomy depends on the results of the initial workup, which includes a liver function panel and right upper quadrant ultrasound (US). US is the standard test for the diagnosis of gallbladder stones, but it is less sensitive for stones in the common bile duct. This is due to the presence of the duodenum adjacent to the distal bile duct and interference of luminal gas with the US image, making it difficult to examine the entire length of the bile duct. Therefore, the sensitivity of US for choledocholithiasis is only 50%, and the presence of choledocholithiasis is usually inferred by a dilated bile duct on US (>6 mm). In some patients, computed tomography (CT) scan of the abdomen is obtained to rule out other causes of jaundice and abdominal pain.

B. The detection of choledocholithiasis on US or CT scan, or the presence of both an elevated bilirubin more than 4 mg/dL and a dilated bile duct is considered a strong predictor of choledocholithiasis. Common bile duct dilation is defined as >6 mm in patients with intact gallbladder, and >8 mm in those who have undergone cholecystectomy. In addition, the clinical suspicion of cholangitis in a patient with gallstones is a strong predictor of choledocholithiasis. If any of these strong predictors of choledocholithiasis is present, then workup should proceed directly with endoscopic retrograde cholangiopancreatography (ERCP) based on the high probability of choledocholithiasis, and the need for biliary decompression in suspected cholangitis.

C. If none of the strong predictors are present but the patient has intermediate probability of choledocholithiasis, then workup can proceed with either endoscopic ultrasound (EUS) or magnetic resonance cholangiopancreatography (MRCP), or proceed with cholecystectomy and intraoperative cholangiogram (IOC) or US. EUS provides high-resolution images of the bile duct without interference by bowel gas or the abdominal wall. It is highly accurate for excluding or confirming choledocholithiasis, with a sensitivity of >95% and specificity of ~97%. Some studies found a higher sensitivity of EUS for choledocholithiasis compared to ERCP. MRCP is a noninvasive

modality that produces highly detailed bile duct and pancreatic duct images with a sensitivity of ~93% and specificity of ~94%. IOC is a procedure performed by the surgeon during cholecystectomy, in which an incision is made into the cystic duct, followed by insertion of a cholangiogram catheter and injection of contrast to delineate biliary anatomy under fluoroscopy. Most studies have found that the sensitivity and specificity of IOC to be greater than 90%. Laparoscopic US is considered an alternative intraoperative method for the detection of choledocholithiasis compared to IOC. A flexible US probe is inserted through the umbilical port and the camera is placed through the epigastric port. The probe is then maneuvered to follow the common bile duct and examine for choledocholithiasis. This technique has 87% sensitivity and 100% specificity for common bile duct stones, but it is not widely available.

D. Patients with positive findings of choledocholithiasis on EUS or MRCP should undergo ERCP for stone extraction and common bile duct clearance. This is followed by cholecystectomy.

E. Patients with positive findings of choledocholithiasis during IOC or US are referred to postoperative ERCP for stone extraction. A less preferred approach is laparoscopic or open bile duct exploration for stone extraction and bile duct clearance.

F. Cases without any predictors of choledocholithiasis are considered low probability for choledocholithiasis and management can proceed with cholecystectomy without further investigations for choledocholithiasis.

BIBLIOGRAPHY

1. ASGE Standards of Practice Committee, Abbas Fehmi SM, Sultan S, et al. ASGE guideline on the role of endoscopy in the evaluation and management of choledocholithiasis. *Gastrointest Endosc.* 2019;89(6):1075-1105. e15.
2. Sleisenger and Fordtran's Gastrointestinal and Liver Disease, 11th Edition, Elsevier, 2021. Chapter 65: Gallstone disease.
3. Hope WW, Fanelli R, Walsh DS, et al. SAGES clinical spotlight review: intraoperative cholangiography. Surg Endosc. 2017;31(5):2007-2016. https://doi.org/10.1007/s00464-016-5320-0.
4. Aziz O, Ashrafian H, Jones C, et al. Laparoscopic ultrasonography versus intra-operative cholangiogram for the detection of common bile duct stones during laparoscopic cholecystectomy: a meta-analysis of diagnostic accuracy. Int J Surg. 2014;12(7):712-719. https://doi.org/10.1016/j.ijsu.2014.05.038.

ALGORITHM 54.1 Flowchart for the workup and management of patients with suspected choledocholithiasis. *CT,* Computed tomography; *CBD,* common bile duct; ERCP, endoscopic retrograde cholangiopancreatography; *EUS,* endoscopic ultrasound; *MRCP,* magnetic resonance cholangiopancreatography; *US,* ultrasound.

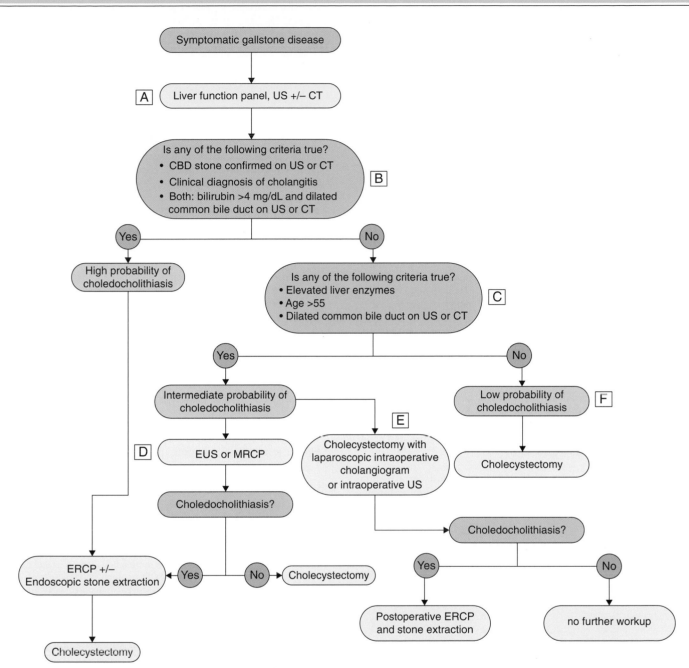

55 Sphincter of Oddi Dysfunction

Emad Qayed

Sphincter of Oddi dysfunction (SOD) refers to the clinical syndrome that occurs due to a noncalculous obstructive process at the sphincter of Oddi (SO). It is caused by stenosis and/or spasm at the level of the sphincter. SOD presents with persistent or recurrent biliary pain following cholecystectomy or with biliary-type pain in patients with an intact gallbladder without cholelithiasis. After cholecystectomy, around 10%–20% of patients experience recurrent pain similar to the pain before cholecystectomy. The most likely cause of this recurrent pain is that the preoperative pain and other symptoms were not related to gallbladder disease. The most likely cause of pain is a disorder of gut–brain interaction (functional pain) such as functional dyspepsia or irritable bowel syndrome. SOD is present in 9%–14% of patients evaluated for postcholecystectomy pain. SOD has been associated with acquired immunodeficiency syndrome (AIDS) cholangiopathy, liver transplant, and chronic opiate use. Less commonly SOD presents with recurrent pancreatitis.

A. The initial evaluation of a patient with biliary-type pain and suspected SOD should include a careful history (biliary pain, pancreatitis, cholecystectomy, human immunodeficiency virus [HIV], opiate use) and physical examination. Laboratory and radiologic workup should be reviewed or ordered including a hepatic panel, HIV test, amylase and lipase levels, liver ultrasound, or cross-sectional imaging (computed tomography [CT] or magnetic resonance imaging [MRI]/ magnetic resonance cholangiopancreatography [MRCP]). Further workup may include evaluation of elevated liver enzymes, and upper endoscopy for abdominal pain.

B. If the patient is found to have choledocholithiasis or structural abnormalities of pancreaticobiliary tree (e.g., biliary stricture, tumor), then the diagnosis is not consistent with SOD, and the underlying condition should be addressed.

C. Patients with biliary pain, dilated common bile duct (CBD), and elevated liver enzymes meet the criteria for type 1 SOD, also referred to as "*sphincter of Oddi stenosis*". The treatment of choice is with endoscopic retrograde cholangiopancreatography (ERCP) and sphincterotomy. This condition has been also called "ampullary stenosis."

D. Patients with biliary pain, and either dilated CBD or elevated liver enzymes, but not both, meet criteria for type 2 SOD, also referred to as "*suspected functional biliary sphincter disorder.*" Supportive criteria for this disorder are normal amylase/lipase and abnormal sphincter of Oddi manometry (SOM). Historically, these patients underwent SOM, and an abnormal SOM was followed by sphincterotomy. However, using SOM to stratify these patients is not a practical approach due to lack of sensitivity in detecting patients who respond to sphincterotomy. In addition, SOM is progressively being abandoned in clinical practice. Patients with type 2 SOD who have significant pain and no other etiology for their symptoms are usually treated by ERCP and empiric sphincterotomy. The response to sphincterotomy is lower than with type 1 SOD; therefore it is important to carefully discuss the risks and benefits of ERCP with these patients. Rectal indomethacin and/or pancreatic stenting should be used to decrease the risk of post-ERCP pancreatitis.

E. The Evaluating Predictors and Interventions in Sphincter of Oddi Dysfunction (EPISOD) trial found that patients who were formerly classified as having SOD type 3 (biliary pain with no CBD dilation and no liver enzymes elevation) do not benefit from empiric sphincterotomy compared to sham intervention. Patients with biliary pain without CBD dilation or liver enzyme elevation are considered to have functional pain, and the term *SOD type 3* has been abandoned. ERCP is not recommended, and these patients should be managed like other functional abdominal pain syndromes.

BIBLIOGRAPHY

1. Yang D, Yachimski P. Cost effective therapy for sphincter of Oddi dysfunction. *Clin Gastroenterol Hepatol.* 2018;16(3):328-330.
2. Sleisenger and Fordtran's Gastrointestinal and Liver Disease, 11th Edition, Elsevier, 2021. Chapter 63, Biliary Tract Motor Function and Dysfunction.
3. Cotton PB, Durkalski V, Romagnuolo J, et al. Effect of endoscopic sphincterotomy for suspected sphincter of Oddi dysfunction on pain-related disability following cholecystectomy: the EPISOD randomized clinical trial. *JAMA.* 2014;311(20):2101-2109. https://doi.org/10.1001/jama.2014.5220.

ALGORITHM 55.1 Flowchart for workup and diagnosis of a patient with suspected sphincter of Oddi dysfunction (*SOD*). *CBC*, Complete blood count; *CT*, computed tomography; *ERCP*, endoscopic retrograde cholangiopancreatography; *HIV*, human immunodeficiency virus; *MRCP*, magnetic resonance cholangiopancreatography; *MRI*, magnetic resonance imaging; *US*, ultrasound.

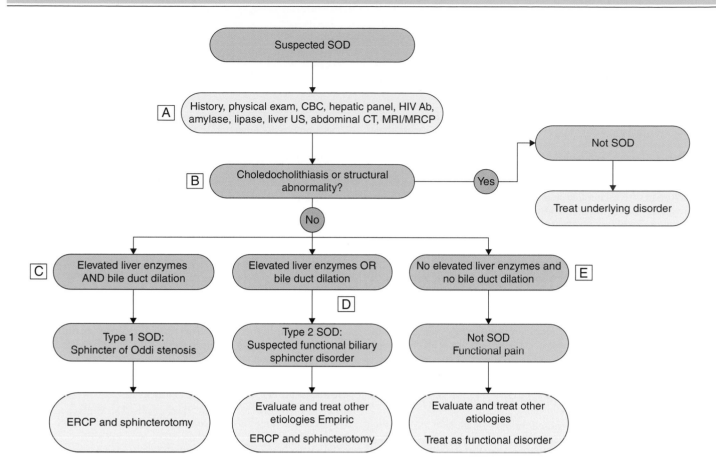

56 Choledochal Cysts

Emad Qayed

Choledochal cysts present as focal or diffuse extrahepatic bile ductal dilatations with varying degrees of intrahepatic dilations. Therefore, they do not represent actual cysts because they are not enclosed epithelialized structures, and more accurately may be referred to as choledochal malformations. Around 80% of choledochal cysts are diagnosed in infants and young children younger than 10 years of age. Infants may present with failure to thrive, jaundice, and abdominal distension. Choledochal cysts in adults may be discovered incidentally, or patients may develop manifestations of biliary obstruction, cholangitis, and pancreatitis. The etiology of these choledochal malformations is not clear, but could be related to congenital weakness of the bile duct wall, or abnormal epithelial proliferation during embryogenesis. Choledochal malformations are associated with anomalous pancreaticobiliary duct union (pancreaticobiliary malunion) in 30%–70% of cases. In this condition, the common bile duct joins the pancreatic duct outside the duodenal wall, forming a long common channel that leads to reflux of pancreatic secretions into the biliary tract. This reflux may lead to progressive injury and dilatation of the bile duct wall. The diagnosis of choledochal cysts is established by ultrasound and confirmed with magnetic resonance cholangiopancreatography (MRCP). Choledochal cysts are associated with increased risk of cholangiocarcinoma (greatest risk is in type 1 and 4 cysts) and their management approach depends on the type and location of cyst.

A. If a choledochal cyst is diagnosed on ultrasound, MRCP should be obtained to confirm the type and location of the cyst and rule out obstructing lesions. Endoscopic ultrasound (EUS) and endoscopic retrograde cholangiopancreatography (ERCP) are complementary tests to evaluate the biliary mucosa if malignancy is suspected. Cholangioscopy can be performed during ERCP to directly examine the biliary mucosa inside the choledochal cyst.

B. Type 1 choledochal cysts present as fusiform dilatation of the extrahepatic bile duct. This dilation could be segmental or diffuse. Management is with cyst excision with Roux-en-Y biliary-enteric reconstruction (hepaticojejunostomy).

C. Type 2 choledochal cysts present as a true diverticulum arising from the bile duct. Management is with simple cyst excision.

D. Type 3 choledochal cyst is also referred to as a *"choledochocele"* and represents dilatation of the distal intraduodenal portion of the bile duct. Management of symptomatic patients is with ERCP and sphincterotomy. Type 3 cysts have low risk of malignancy.

E. Type 4a choledochal cysts present as multiple intra- and extrahepatic bile duct dilatations. Management is with cyst excision and hepaticojejunostomy and segmental hepatectomy of localized intrahepatic liver involvement.

F. Type 4b choledochal cysts present as multiple extrahepatic bile duct dilatations. Management is with simple cyst excision and hepaticojejunostomy.

G. Type 5 choledochal cysts present as single or multiple intrahepatic bile duct dilatations (Caroli disease). Management is with segmental hepatectomy if there is localized disease. However, in diffuse disease, liver transplantation is needed to prevent recurrent episodes of cholangitis and eliminate the risk of cholangiocarcinoma.

BIBLIOGRAPHY

1. Ronnekleiv-Kelly SM, Soares KC, Ejaz A, Pawlik TM. Management of choledochal cysts. *Curr Opin Gastroenterol.* 2016;32(3):225-231.
2. Sleisenger and Fordtran's Gastrointestinal and Liver Disease, 11th Edition, Elsevier, 2021. Chapter 62: Anatomy, Histology, Embryology, Developmental Anomalies, and Pediatric Disorders of the Biliary Tract.
3. Soares KC, Arnaoutakis DJ, Kamel I, et al. Choledochal cysts: presentation, clinical differentiation, and management. *J Am Coll Surg.* 2014;219(6):1167-1180. https://doi.org/10.1016/j.jamcollsurg.2014.04.023.

ALGORITHM 56.1 Flowchart for the workup and management of patients with choledochal cysts, *MRCP*: Magnetic resonance cholangiopancreatography.

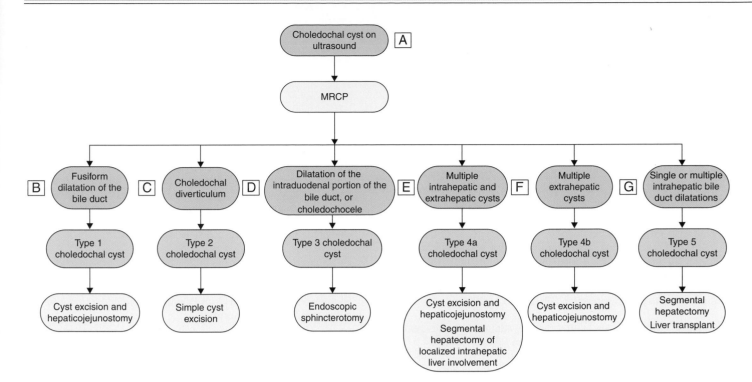

57 Acute Pancreatitis

Emad Qayed

Acute pancreatitis (AP) is defined by meeting two of the following three criteria: (1) abdominal pain typical of AP (e.g., acute onset epigastric, left upper quadrant pain, often radiating to the back); (2) a serum amylase or lipase level ≥3 times the upper limit of normal; and (3) characteristic findings of AP on abdominal imaging.

A. The initial management of AP is critical because it can alter the course of disease and affect the duration of hospitalization. Pancreatic inflammation often leads to the systemic inflammatory response syndrome (SIRS), and persistent SIRS is associated with the development of organ failure (renal, cardiovascular, and pulmonary systems). This organ failure is defined by the latest revision of the Atlanta classification as follows: acute kidney injury (creatinine ≥1.9 mg/dL), hypotension (systolic blood pressure <90 mm Hg, not responsive to fluids), and oxygen desaturation ($[PaO_2/FiO_2]$ <300).

B. Patients without organ failure can be admitted to the general floor and require frequent monitoring and fluid resuscitation. The American Gastroenterological Association suggests judicious goal-directed therapy, in which intravenous (IV) fluids are titrated to clinical and biochemical targets of perfusion such as heart rate, mean arterial pressure, central venous pressure (if available), urine output, blood urea nitrogen concentration, and hematocrit. A recent randomized trial (WATERFALL trial) showed that an aggressive fluid resuscitation regimen led to higher rate of fluid overload and no differences in important clinical outcomes, compared to moderate resuscitation. Due to the increased fluid overload in the aggressive resuscitation group, the trial was stopped early before full recruitment of the planned sample size; however, there was no difference in the incidence of moderately severe or severe pancreatitis between the two groups. Therefore, it is reasonable to give IV fluid bolus only if there are signs of hypovolemia, followed by a moderate fluid infusion rate of 1.5 mL/kg/hour in all patients. If signs of fluid overload develop, then IV fluids should be stopped or decreased.

C. Patients who have signs of organ failure on presentation should be admitted to the intensive care unit (ICU), or at least to an intermediate-care unit (step-down) for close monitoring and meticulous supportive care.

D. Patients who can tolerate oral feeding should be started on an oral diet as tolerated. Those who cannot tolerate oral feeding should be re-evaluated frequently and considered for nasogastric or nasojejunal feeding within 48–72 hours.

E. Patients with rising bilirubin levels should be evaluated for biliary obstruction. Urgent endoscopic retrograde cholangiopancreatography (ERCP) is indicated in cases of acute cholangitis.

F. Patients who are improving and who do not have persistent organ failure are given an oral diet and should be transitioned to oral analgesics. The underlying cause of AP should be addressed. A brief alcohol counseling intervention for patients with alcoholic AP is recommended. Cholecystectomy is recommended before hospital discharge in those with acute gallstone pancreatitis.

G. Patients with AP who are not improving after 48 hours of supportive care, and those with persistent organ failure (severe AP) should be transferred to ICU if they are not already there. Abdominal computed tomography (CT) scan with IV contrast should be performed to evaluate for pancreatic necrosis.

H. Patients who have severe AP with necrosis should receive supportive care, with avoidance of prophylactic antibiotics. Interventions on pancreatic necrosis should be delayed, as possible, beyond 2–4 weeks. However, in patients with concern for infection (e.g., retroperitoneal air), percutaneous drainage should be strongly considered.

I. Patients with persistent symptoms, organ failure, or nutritional failure beyond 2–4 weeks should be considered for drainage and debridement using endoscopic, percutaneous, or minimally invasive surgical approaches. In addition, patients with evidence of infection (e.g., air in necrotic areas on abdominal imaging) should undergo drainage and debridement.

BIBLIOGRAPHY

1. Crockett SD, Wani S, Gardner TB, Falck-Ytter Y, Barkun AN, American Gastroenterological Association Institute Clinical Guidelines Committee. American Gastroenterological Association Institute guideline on initial management of acute pancreatitis. *Gastroenterology*. 2018;154(4):1096-1101.
2. Banks PA, Bollen TL, Dervenis C, et al. Classification of acute pancreatitis--2012: revision of the Atlanta classification and definitions by international consensus. *Gut*. 2013;62(1):102-111.
3. Baron TH, DiMaio CJ, Wang AY, et al. American Gastroenterological Association clinical practice update: management of pancreatic necrosis. *Gastroenterology*. 2020;158(1):67-75. e1.
4. Sleisenger and Fordtran's Gastrointestinal and Liver Disease, 11th Edition, Elsevier, 2021. Chapter 58, Acute pancreatitis.
5. de-Madaria E, Buxbaum JL, Maisonneuve P, et al. Aggressive or moderate fluid resuscitation in acute pancreatitis. *N Engl J Med*. 2022;387(11):989-1000.

ALGORITHM 57.1 Flowchart for the management of acute pancreatitis. *BUN*, Blood urea nitrogen; *CT*, computed tomography; *ERCP*, endoscopic retrograde cholangiopancreatography; *ICU*, intensive care unit; *IV*, intravenous; *NG*, nasogastric; *NJ*, nasojejunal; *NPO*, nil per os; *TG*, triglycerides.

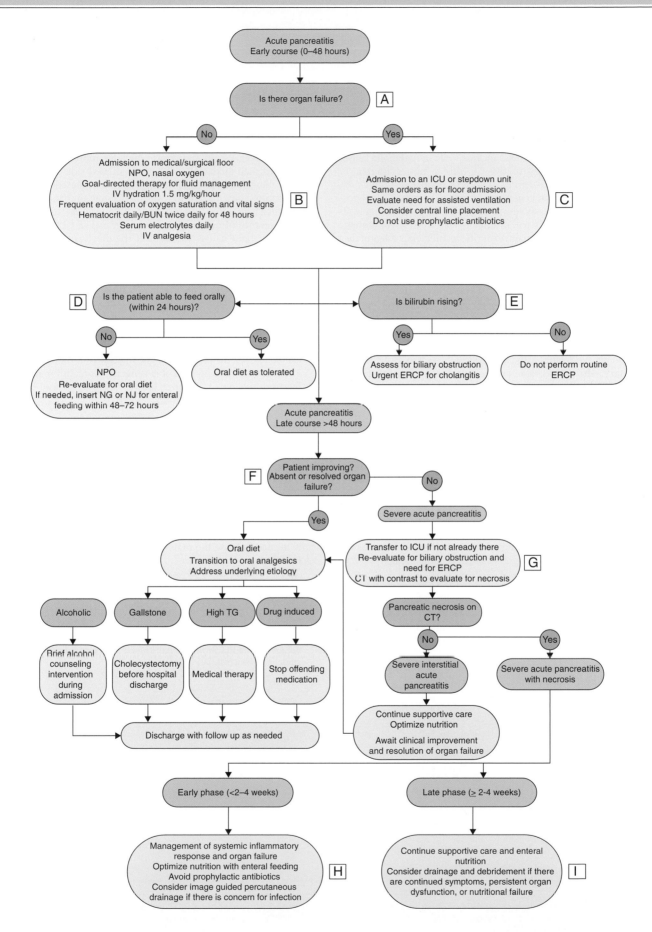

58 Chronic Pancreatitis

Vaishali Patel

The term *"chronic pancreatitis"* (CP) refers to a chronic inflammation and fibrosis of the pancreas that leads to the destruction of ductal, exocrine, and endocrine tissue. Long-standing heavy alcohol use is the most common etiology of CP. Other causes include toxic or metabolic causes (smoking, hyperlipidemia), obstructive CP (due to tumor, trauma, or congenital anomalies such as annular pancreas or pancreas divisum), autoimmune pancreatitis, and genetic mutations. A complete list of possible etiologies for CP is presented in Box 58.1. Any process that leads to recurrent acute pancreatitis will eventually lead to CP. Symptomatic CP leads to chronic abdominal pain, exocrine insufficiency (steatorrhea and malabsorption), and endocrine insufficiency (diabetes mellitus). In some patients, CP does not lead to abdominal pain, and the disease is discovered incidentally or as part of the workup of steatorrhea.

A. In patients suspected to have CP, a thorough history and physical examination should be performed. It is especially important to assess for risk factors for CP including exposure history (most commonly chronic alcohol or tobacco exposure), family history of pancreatitis or known genetic syndromes associated with CP (such as cystic fibrosis or hereditary pancreatitis), and number of prior episodes of acute pancreatitis. Additionally, it is important to assess the nature of symptoms, including character of abdominal pain, presence of steatorrhea, symptoms suggestive of vitamin deficiency, malabsorption, or weight loss.

B. A key part of CP diagnosis is documenting the presence of the typical morphologic features of the disease. Cross-sectional imaging with computed tomography (CT) or magnetic resonance imaging (MRI) is the initial diagnostic test of choice to evaluate the morphology of the pancreas. Morphologic features of CP include pancreatic atrophy, ductal strictures and dilatation of variable degrees, ductal stones, and parenchymal calcification. In advanced CP cases, the pancreatic duct is severely dilated with alternating strictures (the chain-of-lakes appearance). If typical morphologic changes of the pancreas are seen, then the diagnosis of CP is confirmed.

C. Endoscopic ultrasound (EUS) is performed if the diagnosis of CP is still unclear after performing cross-sectional imaging, and if there is high clinical suspicion of CP with subtle morphologic changes. There are several endosonographic criteria and scoring systems for EUS-based diagnosis of CP; however, current evidence does not support using EUS alone to establish the diagnosis of CP. Therefore the diagnosis of CP based on EUS findings should be combined with the presence of clinical features and risk factors of CP.

D. In rare circumstances when CT, MRI, or EUS is not diagnostic of CP, and the clinical suspicion of CP remains high, secretin-enhanced magnetic resonance cholangiopancreatography (s-MRCP) may be used to evaluate the pancreatic duct for more subtle morphologic changes such as ductal strictures or dilated side branches. If available, pancreatic function testing with tube-based secretin test or endoscopic-based secretin test can evaluate for exocrine pancreatic insufficiency (EPI). Other tests include fecal fat and fecal elastase. The presence of EPI supports the diagnosis of CP, but there is controversy about its use to establish the diagnosis of CP. EPI can be present without CP, but is important to recognize in patients with CP so that it can be appropriately treated. The presence of EPI alone has low sensitivity to make the diagnosis of CP, as most patients with CP do not have EPI. EPI usually manifests following the loss of >90% of pancreatic function. Symptoms of EPI may include steatorrhea, azotorrhea, vitamin deficiency, and weight loss. A 72-hour fecal fat measurement is considered the gold standard for diagnosis, however may prove inconvenient for patients. Reduced levels of fecal elastase can be used as the primary diagnostic test with moderate sensitivity. The cutoff of <200 µg/g stool is generally used, but may have a high false positive result. A lower level of <100 µg/g stool has a higher specificity but lower sensitivity.

E. In young patients with clinical suspicion of CP of unclear etiology, genetic testing for CP mutations is recommended. Examples of genetic polymorphisms implicated in CP include PRSS1 (cationic trypsinogen gene), CPA1 (carboxypeptidase A1 gene), CEL (carboxyl ester lipase), SPINK1 (serine protein inhibitor Kazal type 1), CTRC (chymotrypsin C), and CFTR (cystic fibrosis transmembrane conductance regulator). In patients with high clinical suspicion of CP, EUS and fine needle aspiration/core biopsy can be considered to perform a histologic examination of the pancreas. This is rarely needed because the majority of CP cases are diagnosed based on morphologic features.

BIBLIOGRAPHY

1. Gardner TB, Adler DG, Forsmark CE, et al. ACG Clinical Guideline: chronic pancreatitis. American Journal. *Gastroenterology*. 2020;115:322-339.
2. Conwell DL, Lee LS, Yadav D, et al. American Pancreatic Association Practice Guidelines in Chronic Pancreatitis: evidence-based report on diagnostic guidelines. *Pancreas*. 2014;43(8):1143-1162.

ALGORITHM 58.1 Flowchart for the diagnosis of chronic pancreatitis. *CT*, Computed tomography; *ERCP*, endoscopic retrograde cholangiopancreatography; *EUS*, endoscopic ultrasound; *FNA*, fine needle aspiration; *MRCP*, magnetic resonance cholangiopancreatography; *MRI*, magnetic resonance imaging; *PTC*, percutaneous cholangiography.

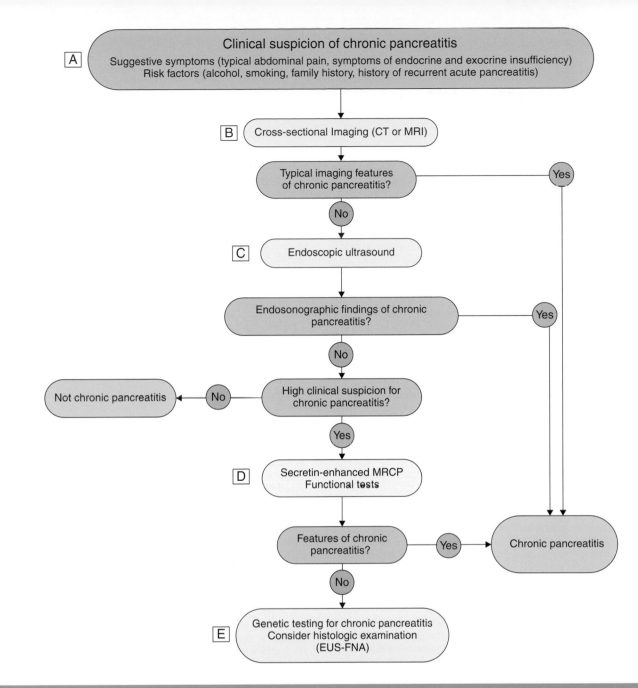

A. Clinical suspicion of chronic pancreatitis

Suggestive symptoms (typical abdominal pain, symptoms of endocrine and exocrine insufficiency)
Risk factors (alcohol, smoking, family history, history of recurrent acute pancreatitis)

B. Cross-sectional Imaging (CT or MRI)

Typical imaging features of chronic pancreatitis? — Yes → Chronic pancreatitis

No

C. Endoscopic ultrasound

Endosonographic findings of chronic pancreatitis? — Yes → Chronic pancreatitis

No

High clinical suspicion for chronic pancreatitis? — No → Not chronic pancreatitis

Yes

D. Secretin-enhanced MRCP
Functional tests

Features of chronic pancreatitis? — Yes → Chronic pancreatitis

No

E. Genetic testing for chronic pancreatitis
Consider histologic examination
(EUS-FNA)

BOX 58.1 CLASSIFICATION OF CHRONIC PANCREATITIS

TOXIC-METABOLIC

Alcohol

Tobacco
Hypercalcemia
Hypertrigycia Chronic renal failure

IDIOPATHIC

Tropical calcific pancreatitis
Fibrocalculous pancreatic diabetes
Early-onset idiopathic
Late-onset idiopathic

RECURRENT AND SEVERE ACUTE PANCREATITIS

Postnecrotic (after severe necrotizing pancreatitis)
Vascular disease/ischemia

OBSTRUCTIVE

Benign pancreatic duct obstruction Traumatic stricture
Stricture after severe acute pancreatitis
Ampullary obstruction
Sphincter of Oddi stenosis

Celiac disease
Crohn's disease
Duodenal wall cyst
Pancreas divisum

GENETIC

Autosomal dominant
  Hereditary pancreatitis (PRSS1 mutations)
Autosomal recessive or modifier genes
  CFTR mutations
  SPINK1 mutations
  Chymotrypsin C mutations
  Claudin mutations

Calcium-sensing receptor gene
Carboxy ethyl lipase
Others

AUTOIMMUNE PANCREATITIS

IgG4-related systemic disease, type 1

IgG4-related systemic disease, type 2

RECURRENT AND SEVERE ACUTE PANCREATITIS

Malignant pancreatic duct obstruction
  Ampullary carcinoma
  Duodenal carcinoma
  Pancreatic ductal adenocarcinoma
  Intraductal papillary mucinous neoplasm

ASYMPTOMATIC PANCREATIC FIBROSIS

Chronic alcohol use
Old age
Chronic kidney disease
Diabetes mellitus

Previous radiotherapy

Ig, Immunoglobulin G; *PRSS1*, protease serine 1 gene; *SPINK1*, serine protease inhibitor, Kazal type 1 gene.

59 Pancreatic Cysts

Vaishali Patel

Pancreatic cysts have been diagnosed more frequently in recent years due to the increased use of abdominal cross-sectional imaging and the improved diagnostic quality of these studies. Various types of pancreatic cysts exist, but only some have malignant potential, most notably intraductal papillary mucinous neoplasms (IPMNs) and mucinous cystic neoplasms (MCNs). While the overall risk of malignancy at the time of diagnosis for all pancreatic cysts is <1% (with a yearly conversion rate of <0.5%), available retrospective data suggest that IPMNs have a higher risk of developing high-grade dysplasia or pancreatic cancer (overall risk estimated to be 2.8%, or 0.72% per year). Low-risk IPMNs have been shown to have an approximately 3% pooled cumulative incidence of high-grade dysplasia or pancreatic cancer at 5 years. In contrast, the cumulative incidence in high-risk IPMNs (with an associated mural nodule or pancreatic main duct dilatation) is estimated to be 9.8% at 5 years.

The primary treatment for a pancreatic cyst is surgical resection when indicated. Given the invasiveness, cost, morbidity (30%), and mortality (2.1%) associated with this, caution is recommended with regards to proceeding with surveillance of cysts. Large cysts with worrisome features are frequently found in older patients with multiple comorbidities; however, individual life expectancy and candidacy for surgery should be considered when deciding the optimal evaluation and management of a pancreatic cystic lesion. Patients who are not candidates for surgery or oncologic management should not undergo pancreatic cyst surveillance, regardless of cyst size.

Magnetic resonance imaging (MRI) with magnetic resonance cholangiopancreatography (MRCP) allows for noninvasive accurate characterization of pancreatic cysts, as well as any communication of the cystic lesion with the main duct or side branches (important because side-branch IPMNs have a lower risk of progression cancer). It is therefore the test of choice for both initial diagnosis and surveillance. For example, serous cystadenomas typically have a microcystic appearance on imaging with a central stellate scar. For patients who cannot undergo MRI, alternative modes of imaging are pancreatic-protocol computed tomography (CT) or endoscopic ultrasound (EUS). These imaging studies alone provide 40%–50% accuracy in determining cyst type; however, in cases where the diagnosis is indeterminate, it is recommended that EUS with fine needle aspiration (FNA) be performed for cyst fluid analysis (fluid amylase and carcinoembryonic antigen [CEA] levels) to determine cyst type as this impacts their management. IPMNs and MCNs have high CEA levels and variable or high amylase levels. Pseudocysts and serous cystadenomas generally have low CEA levels. Inflammatory pseudocysts will have a high amylase level. Patients who have a clinical history and imaging consistent with an acute or chronic inflammatory pancreatic pseudocyst should undergo appropriate management of the fluid collection, rather than long-term imaging surveillance. Additionally, depending on their clinical status, patients with lesions that have typical features of a cyst with low risk of malignant transformation (such as serous cystadenomas) should defer further surveillance.

A. Patients with cystic lesions presumed to be MCNs or IPMNs should be evaluated for the presence of concerning clinical and radiologic features.

B. If any concerning feature is present, patients should undergo multidisciplinary evaluation for EUS with FNA sampling.

C. If the cytology results are consistent with high-grade dysplasia or malignancy, then referral for surgical resection is appropriate.

D. If there are no findings concerning for malignancy on EUS/FNA, then surveillance with MRI and/or EUS is recommended every 3–6 months. If size remains stable, then surveillance intervals can be lengthened.

E. If no concerning features are present, then surveillance with MRI based on cyst size is recommended. Cysts that increase in size more than 3 mm/year require further evaluation with EUS/FNA.

BIBLIOGRAPHY

1. Elta GH, Enestvedt BK, Sauer BG, et al. ACG clinical guideline: diagnosis and management of pancreatic cysts. *Am J Gastroenterol.* 2018;113(4):464-479.
2. Buerlein R, Shami V. Management of pancreatic cysts and guidelines: what the gastroenterologist needs to know. *Therapeutic Advances in Gastrointestinal Endoscopy.* 2021;14:26317745211045769.

ALGORITHM 59.1 Flowchart for the workup and diagnosis of a patient with intrapapillary mucinous tumor or mucinous cystic neoplasm. *EUS,* Endoscopic ultrasound; *FNA,* fine needle aspiration; *IPMN,* intrapapillary mucinous neoplasm; *MRI,* magnetic resonance imaging.

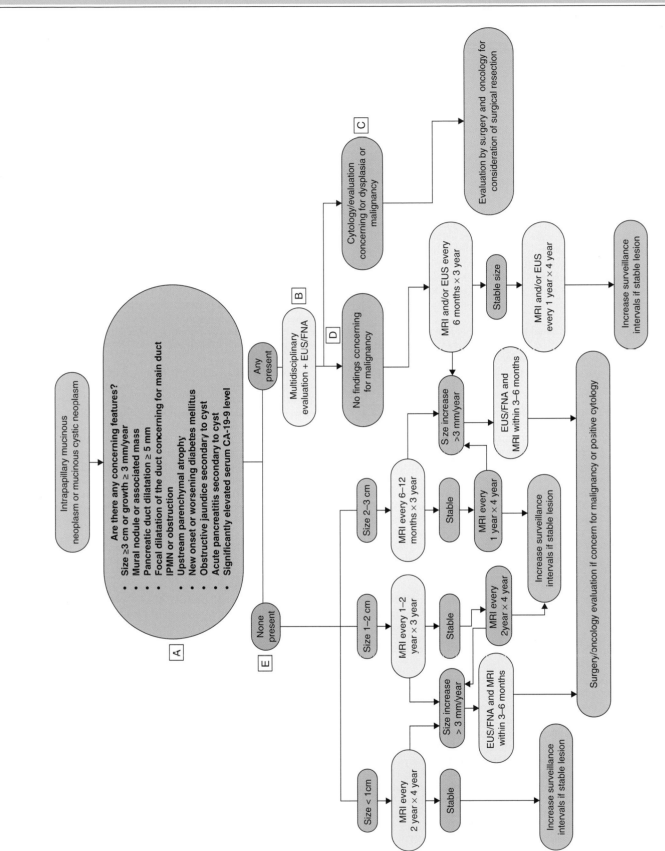

Intrapapillary mucinous neoplasm or mucinous cystic neoplasm

A

Are there any concerning features?
- **Size ≥3 cm or growth ≥ 3 mm/year**
- **Mural nodule or associated mass**
- **Pancreatic duct dilatation ≥ 5 mm**
- **Focal dilatation of the duct concerning for main duct IPMN or obstruction**
- **Upstream parenchymal atrophy**
- **New onset or worsening diabetes mellitus**
- **Obstructive jaundice secondary to cyst**
- **Acute pancreatitis secondary to cyst**
- **Significantly elevated serum CA-19-9 level**

Any present

B Multidisciplinary evaluation + EUS/FNA

C Cytology/evaluation concerning for dysplasia or malignancy

Evaluation by surgery and oncology for consideration of surgical resection

D No findings concerning for malignancy

MRI and/or EUS every 6 months × 3 year → Stable size → MRI and/or EUS every 1 year × 4 year → Increase surveillance intervals if stable lesion

Size increase >3 mm/year → EUS/FNA and MRI within 3–6 months

E None present

Size < 1cm → MRI every 2 year × 4 year → Stable → Increase surveillance intervals if stable lesion

Size 1–2 cm → MRI every 1–2 year × 3 year → Stable → MRI every 2year × 4 year → Increase surveillance intervals if stable lesion

Size increase > 3 mm/year → EUS/FNA and MRI within 3–6 months

Size 2–3 cm → MRI every 6–12 months × 3 year → Stable → MRI every 1 year × 4 year → Increase surveillance intervals if stable lesion

Size increase >3 mm/year → EUS/FNA and MRI within 3–6 months

Surgery/oncology evaluation if concern for malignancy or positive cytology

60 Celiac Disease

Nikrad Shahnavaz

Celiac disease is a chronic, immune-mediated enteropathy that is triggered by dietary gluten in a genetically predisposed (HLA DQ2/DQ8) individual. The prevalence of celiac disease in the United States is about 0.7%, although the majority of cases are undiagnosed. Symptoms, signs, and laboratory findings of celiac disease vary with the extent and severity of the intestinal involvement as well as the characteristics of the patient.

A. Celiac disease should be suspected in asymptomatic patients with a family history of celiac disease or in patients with associated disorders, such as type 1 diabetes, Hashimoto thyroiditis, Down syndrome, iron deficiency anemia, transaminitis, peripheral neuropathy, osteoporosis, or infertility. Gastrointestinal manifestations of celiac disease include bloating, diarrhea, steatorrhea, abdominal pain, or malabsorption.

B. Diagnosis of celiac disease could be challenging in patients who are already on gluten-free diet. The first step in these patients is to test for HLA DQ2/DQ8. A negative test for both haplotypes will rule out the diagnosis of celiac disease and preclude the need for gluten challenge or other testing.

C. Gluten challenge should be started with caution, as in rare cases, patients could be severely sensitive to gluten. The low-dose gluten challenge (3 g daily) is effective in causing histologic and serologic changes without triggering intolerable symptoms. A biopsy could be performed after 2 weeks but serologic testing is more sensitive 4–6 weeks after the onset of the gluten challenge.

D. The sensitivity and specificity of tissue transglutaminase (TTG) immunoglobulin (Ig)A antibody are both around 95% when the test is performed in patients on gluten-containing diet. Up to 5% of patients with celiac disease may have immunoglobulin A (IgA) deficiency; therefore serum IgA level should also be checked along with TTG-IgA antibody.

E. In patients with very low serum IgA levels, testing for TTG-IgA could give a false negative result. TTG-IgG antibody or deamidated gliadin peptide (DGP) IgG antibody should be measured. In general, there is no use of checking gliadin IgG antibody due to its low sensitivity and specificity.

F. Biopsy of the small intestine during upper endoscopy is the gold standard test to confirm diagnosis. At least four biopsies from the second portion of the duodenum and two biopsies from the duodenal bulb should be obtained to increase the sensitivity of the test. Modified Marsh classification of histologic findings is used to describe the severity of the small intestine involvement, which ranges between Marsh 1 (increased intraepithelial lymphocytes) and Marsh 3 C (total villous atrophy). Increased intraepithelial cells and villous atrophy in the duodenum could also be seen in nonceliac causes such as nonsteroidal antiinflammatory drugs (NSAIDs) use, *Helicobacter pylori* infection, small intestinal bacterial overgrowth, Crohn's disease, human immunodeficiency virus (HIV) enteropathy, lymphoma, or common variable immunodeficiency (CVID).

G. After 3 to 6 months of strict gluten-free diet, the expectation is to witness significant improvement in symptoms, decrease in antibody titers, and improvement of nutritional deficiencies.

H. Repeat endoscopy is recommended with small intestinal biopsies and measurement of serum antibody titers after 1 year of strict gluten-free diet to confirm the expected response to treatment.

I. Strict avoidance of gluten in the diet is a challenging task as many hidden sources of gluten are found in food products. Important questions to ask the patient when checking compliance with the gluten-free diet include asking about intentional intake of gluten, and about the patient's confidence in avoiding gluten intake when dining out. Most physicians do not have adequate knowledge or dedicated time to counsel patients about diet during clinic encounters. Registered dietitians are essential to advise and educate the patients on how to maintain a strict gluten-free diet and to provide healthy alternatives to gluten in their diet.

J. Nonresponsive celiac disease is a clinical diagnosis defined by the persistence of typical symptoms, signs, serologic, or histologic abnormalities of celiac disease despite adherence to a gluten-free diet for at least 6–12 months. The first step is to exclude accidental ingestion of gluten in the diet. The next step is to confirm the diagnosis of celiac disease by repeating small intestinal biopsies. If the enteropathy has healed, other etiologies such as lactose/fructose intolerance, irritable bowel syndrome, small intestinal bacterial overgrowth, pancreatic insufficiency, or microscopic colitis should be considered. If enteropathy has not changed, alternative causes of a celiac-like enteropathy including CVID, tropical sprue, giardiasis, Crohn's disease, or HIV enteropathy should be ruled out.

K. Refractory celiac disease is defined as persistent villous atrophy and malabsorption despite a confirmed gluten-free diet for at least 1 year. It is divided into type 1 (less severe with normal intraepithelial lymphocytes) and type 2 (more aggressive disease with abnormal, oligoclonal mucosal T-cell population). Type 2 can progress to enteropathy-associated T-cell lymphoma or ulcerative jejunitis.

BIBLIOGRAPHY

1. Lebwohl B, Green PHR. Celiac disease. Sleisenger and Fordtran's Gastrointestinal and Liver Disease. 11th Edition, 2020.
2. Rubio-Tapia A, Hill ID, Kelly CP, Calderwood AH, Murray JA. American College of Gastroenterology. ACG clinical guidelines: diagnosis and management of celiac disease. *Am J Gastroenterol.* 2013;108(5):656-676.
3. Raiteri A, Granito A, Giamperoli A, Catenaro T, Negrini G, Tovoli F. Current guidelines for the management of celiac disease: a systematic review with comparative analysis. *World J Gastroenterol.* 2022;28(1):154-175.
4. Husby S, Murray JA, Katzka DA. AGA clinical practice update on diagnosis and monitoring of celiac disease-changing utility of serology and histologic measures: expert review. *Gastroenterology.* 2019;156(4):885-889.
5. Leffler DA, Dennis M, Edwards George JB, et al. A simple validated gluten-free diet adherence survey for adults with celiac disease. *Clin Gastroenterol Hepatol.* 2009;7(5):530 536.e5362. https://doi.org/10.1016/j.cgh.2008.12.032.

ALGORITHM 60.1 Flowchart for the diagnosis and treatment of celiac disease. *DGP,* Deamidated gliadin peptide; *HLA,* human leukocyte antigen; *IgA,* immunoglobulin A; *TTG,* tissue transglutaminase.

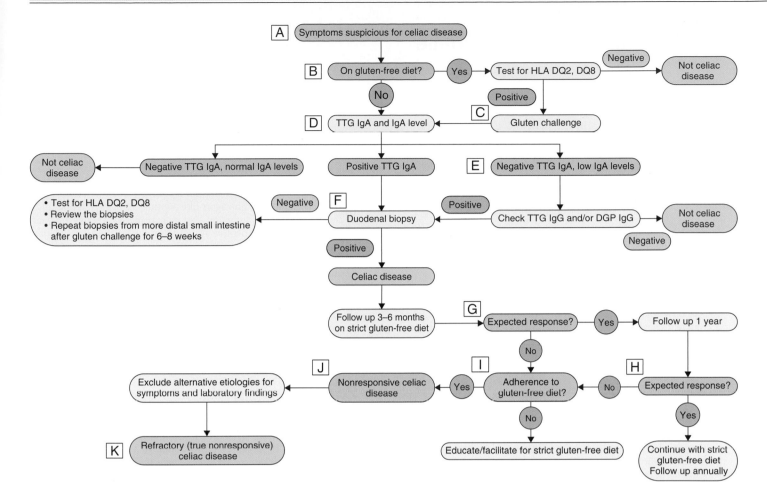

61 Short Bowel Syndrome

Nikrad Shahnavaz

A residual small intestinal length of 200 cm or less meets criteria for short bowel syndrome (SBS). The length of residual bowel is measured at the time of surgery from the duodenojejunal flexure to the ileocecal junction, the site of any enterocolonic anastomosis, or to the endostomy. Based on the presence or absence of residual colon, SBS can be classified into three groups: (1) end-jejunostomy; (2) jejunocolonic anastomosis (jejunum anastomosed to partial colon); and (3) jejunoileocolonic anastomosis (keeping the entire colon and ileocecal valve).

A. If possible, end-jejunostomy anatomy should be converted to jejunocolonic or jejunoileocolonic anatomy, by restoring continuity with any remaining small bowel or colon. This will improve overall prognosis and quality of life.

B. Patients with intact colon and residual small intestinal length of 100 cm or with hemicolectomy and residual small intestinal length of 150 cm can usually meet their nutrition and hydration requirements without parenteral support.

C. Patients with SBS who do not require parenteral support are treated with oral rehydration solutions and their electrolytes should be monitored closely. The use of antisecretory drugs like proton pump inhibitors, histamine-2 receptor antagonists, and less frequently octreotide, is beneficial in reducing the production of a variety of gastrointestinal secretions in these patients. Antidiarrheals, such as loperamide, diphenoxylate with atropine, codeine, and tincture of opium, work mainly to reduce intestinal motility and intestinal secretion. Compensatory hyperphagia with five to six meals during the day is essential. In patients with a colon, a diet with high complex carbohydrate, low fat, low oxalate, and addition of medium-chain triglycerides (MCTs) is recommended.

D. Tunneled central venous catheters are preferred for long-term parenteral support as opposed to peripherally inserted central venous catheters because of the lower risk of thrombosis and less issues related to self-administration of parenteral nutrition. After initiation, parenteral nutrition should be adjusted based on the patient's fluid, electrolyte, energy, protein, and micronutrient needs.

E. About half of adults with SBS can be weaned completely from parenteral support within 5 years of diagnosis. Optimizing oral diet and fluid intake as well as aggressive use of antidiarrheal and antisecretory medications may help to achieve this goal.

F. In selected patients with SBS who have not been able to achieve enteral independence despite optimization of diet and medical management, recombinant glucagon-like peptide-2 (GLP-2), teduglutide as daily subcutaneous injection, can be considered. Teduglutide can improve intestinal absorptive function and allow weaning of parenteral nutrition in these patients. This drug may increase the risk of gastrointestinal malignancies including colon cancer, so patients need to be screened closely by colonoscopy during therapy. The role of surgical intervention in patients with SBS is limited to recruiting unused distal bowel, specific lengthening and tapering operations, or slowing down gut transit.

G. The indications for small intestinal transplantation include parenteral support–dependent SBS complicated by progressive liver disease, significant fluid losses and severe dehydration despite appropriate medical management, thrombosis of two central veins, a single episode of fungemia, a single episode of bacterial sepsis with shock, and two lifetime episodes of catheter sepsis. With improved techniques and optimized immunosuppressive regimens, reported survival and nutritional autonomy after small intestinal transplantation have increased to about 18 years in recent years. On the other hand, late referral for small intestinal transplantation often requires addition of liver transplant and may result in a less optimal outcome.

BIBLIOGRAPHY

1. Buchman AL Short bowel syndrome. Sleisenger and Fordtran's Gastrointestinal and Liver Disease. 11th Edition, Elsevier, 2020.
2. DiBaise JK, Iyer K, Rubio-Tapia A. AGA clinical practice update on management of short bowel syndrome: expert review. *Clin Gastroenterol Hepatol.* 2022;S1542-3565(22):00561-005614.

ALGORITHM 61.1 Management of short bowel syndrome. *GLP-2,* Glucagon-like peptide-2; *PS,* parenteral support.

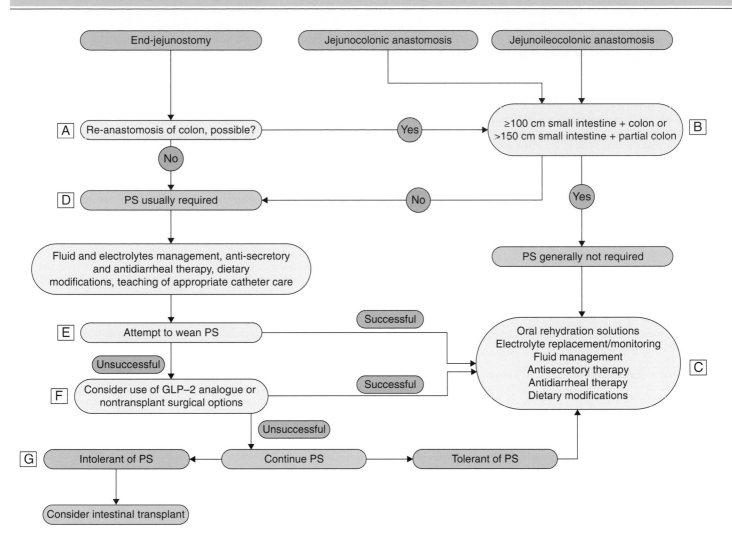

62 Microscopic Colitis

Nikrad Shahnavaz

Microscopic colitis is a common cause of chronic watery diarrhea with characteristic histologic features in the absence of endoscopic or radiologic abnormalities of the colon. It is most commonly diagnosed in older women, generally between the ages of 50 and 70 years. Microscopic colitis has been associated with autoimmune disorders such as type 1 diabetes, celiac disease, and autoimmune thyroiditis. Lymphocytic colitis and collagenous colitis are two variants of microscopic colitis based on histologic findings with similar clinical presentations and treatment. In both diseases, the lamina propria contains a mixed inflammatory infiltrate consisting mainly of lymphocytes and plasma cells. Lymphocytic colitis has intraepithelial lymphocytosis (≥20 intraepithelial lymphocytes per 100 surface epithelial cells). Collagenous colitis has less prominent intraepithelial lymphocytosis, but has a characteristic finding of a thick sub-epithelial collagen band (>10 μm, compared to normal of <5 μm). There is no evidence to suggest that microscopic colitis increases the risk of colon cancer or inflammatory bowel disease. The goal of the treatment is to control the diarrhea and reduce the significant burden on quality of life and healthcare costs.

A. The first step in the management is to identify and discontinue any medication or dietary factor that might cause or exacerbate diarrhea and microscopic colitis. This includes medications such as nonsteroidal antiinflammatory drugs (NSAIDs), selective serotonin reuptake inhibitors, proton pump inhibitors, H2 receptor antagonist, lisinopril, statins, and bisphosphonates. Furthermore, smoking, excessive consumption of artificial sweeteners, or dairy products should be avoided. Cessation of a potential culprit can result in improvement or even resolution of the diarrhea in some patients. However, majority of the patients with microscopic colitis will require active treatment.

B. In patients with mild disease (less than three bowel movements daily and no watery diarrhea), antidiarrheal medications such as diphenoxylate or loperamide may be sufficient to control the diarrhea.

C. For patients with moderate symptoms (three to five loose/watery stool daily), or if antidiarrheal medications alone are unsuccessful, bismuth subsalicylate at a larger dose of three tablets (262 mg each) three times daily can be effective especially in older patients. Long-term use of high-dose bismuth subsalicylate is associated with neurotoxicity and is not recommended.

D. For cases refractory to antidiarrheal and bismuth, or for those with severe diarrhea (more than five loose and watery stools daily), budesonide is recommended. Induction dose for budesonide is 9 mg once daily for 8 weeks, and then can be tapered and discontinued over the course of 4 weeks.

E. Relapse after discontinuation of budesonide is seen in 60%–80% of the patients. Risk factors for steroid dependency include a longer duration of illness before budesonide therapy and more severe diarrhea at baseline.

F. In patients with relapse after discontinuation of budesonide, maintenance therapy should be considered. Common practice is to restart with budesonide 6 mg daily, then taper to the lowest effective dose such as 3 mg daily or every other day to maintain control of diarrhea.

G. True microscopic colitis usually responds to budesonide. Therefore in refractory cases, the first step is to rule out alternative or concomitant diagnoses including celiac disease, small intestinal bacterial overgrowth, bile acid diarrhea, or drug-induced microscopic colitis with persistent exposure to the offending medication.

H. In patients with microscopic colitis refractory to budesonide, bile acid binders such as cholestyramine may be useful as single-agent or adjuvant therapy with budesonide, although the available data supporting their efficacy are limited.

I. For refractory and severe cases of microscopic colitis, prednisone or prednisolone could be considered. However, they are associated with more systemic side effects and higher risk of relapse after withdrawal.

J. Immunomodulators such as thiopurines, methotrexate, or biologic therapy with infliximab could be used in steroid-resistant severe cases, although there are only case reports and small case series to support these treatments.

K. Surgical options such as ileostomy (with or without colectomy) or ileal pouch-anal anastomosis are rarely considered in medication-refractory cases of microscopic colitis with disabling symptoms.

BIBLIOGRAPHY

1. Pardi DS, Cotter TG. Other diseases of the colon. Sleisenger and Fordtran's Gastrointestinal and Liver Disease, 11th Edition, 2020.
2. Pardi DS. Diagnosis and management of microscopic colitis. *Am J Gastroenterol.* 2017;112(1):78-85.

ALGORITHM 62.1 Management of microscopic colitis.

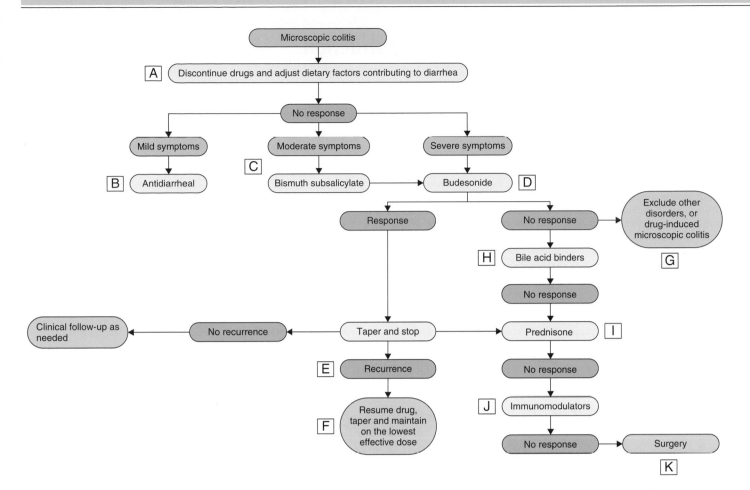

63 Acute Colonic Pseudo-Obstruction

Srikrishna Patnana

Acute colonic pseudo-obstruction (ACPO), also known as *Ogilvie syndrome*, refers to acute massive distension of the colon in the absence of mechanical obstruction. ACPO is generally attributed to alteration in the autonomous nervous system innervation of the colon. Most patients who develop ACPO are elderly with multiple comorbidities who are immobilized in hospital because of severe illness, surgery, or trauma. Conditions associated with ACPO include: trauma; pneumonia; sepsis; myocardial infarction; heart failure; orthopedic, gynecologic, and abdominal surgery; and neurologic disease such as Parkinson disease, spinal cord disease, and multiple sclerosis. Other associated medical conditions include metabolic derangements, malignancy, respiratory failure, and renal failure. Patients typically develop abdominal distension over a few days, along with abdominal pain, nausea, and vomiting.

A. The initial steps in the management of ACPO are to perform a comprehensive history and physical examination to rule out colonic obstruction and complications of ACPO (ischemia and perforation), and to identify any underlying etiology for colonic ileus. Although abdominal x-ray and contrast enema can be performed to diagnose the former, computerized tomography (CT) scan of the abdomen/pelvis is usually done to exclude obstruction and/or perforation.

B. If perforation or peritonitis is present, the patient needs surgical intervention.

C. If mechanical obstruction is diagnosed, treatment may involve surgery or endoscopy depending on the etiology. Flexible sigmoidoscopy is performed for sigmoid detorsion in cases of sigmoid volvulus.

D. Once colonic obstruction, ischemia, and perforation are excluded, the next step in the management of ACPO depends on cecal diameter. Complications of ACPO are unusual with a cecal diameter <12 cm. The risk of ischemia or perforation is 0% with cecal diameter <12 cm, 7% with cecal diameter 12–14 cm, and 23% with cecal diameter >14 cm.

E. If cecal diameter is <12 cm, supportive measures should be instituted for the next 48–72 hours with close monitoring (with examination, laboratory tests, and abdominal x-ray). These include correction of electrolyte abnormalities, ambulation, bowel rest, decompression with nasogastric and rectal tubes, and minimization or avoidance of narcotics and anticholinergic agents.

F. If there is no improvement or worsening of cecal distension to a diameter of >12 cm, neostigmine can be used in the absence of contraindications. Absolute contraindications for its use are intestinal or urinary obstruction. Relative contraindications are bradycardia,

asthma, renal insufficiency, recent myocardial infarction, and acidosis. Neostigmine is an acetylcholinesterase inhibitor, which leads to increased parasympathetic activity. Therefore patients need continuous cardiopulmonary monitoring with access to 0.5 to 1 mg intravenous (IV) atropine in case symptomatic bradycardia develops.

G. Neostigmine is usually administered at a dose of 2 mg IV over 3–5 minutes. It is effective in 85%–95% of patients. If there is no response or partial response, it can be repeated within 2–4 hours and the response rate is 40%–100%. Although neostigmine is usually given as an IV bolus, it can also be given subcutaneously or as a continuous infusion (0.4–0.8 mg/hour), which may lead to better response and fewer side effects.

H. Colonoscopic decompression is performed if there are contraindications to neostigmine use, or if there is no response to neostigmine. It is important to rule out perforation with imaging prior to colonoscopy especially in the presence of severe abdominal tenderness and leukocytosis. Colonoscopy should be performed in an unprepared colon, with water infusion, and minimal carbon dioxide insufflation, and the endoscope should be advanced at least to distal transverse colon with extensive suctioning. Colon decompression tube placement should be considered especially when repeat colonoscopies are performed for recurrent symptoms.

I. If ACPO does not respond to all the aforementioned measures, further treatment options include cecostomy or subtotal colectomy. Surgery is associated with increased morbidity and mortality and should be considered as a last resort except when ACPO is complicated by ischemia or perforation.

J. Once ACPO responds to treatment, daily polyethylene glycol therapy for 1 week is recommended to prevent recurrence of the disease.

BIBLIOGRAPHY

1. Alavi K, Poylin V, Davids JS, et al. The American Society of Colon and Rectal Surgeons clinical practice guidelines for the management of colonic volvulus and acute colonic pseudo-obstruction. *Dis Colon Rectum.* 2021;64(9):1046-1057.
2. Naveed M, Jamil LH, Fujii-Lau LL, et al. American Society for Gastrointestinal Endoscopy guideline on the role of endoscopy in the management of acute colonic pseudo-obstruction and colonic volvulus [published correction appears in *Gastrointest Endosc.* 2020;91(3):721]. *Gastrointest Endosc.* 2020;91(2):228-235.
3. Sleisenger and Fordtran's Gastrointestinal and Liver Disease, 11th Edition, Elsevier, 2021. Chapter 24: Ileus and Pseudo-Obstruction Syndromes.

ALGORITHM 63.1 Flow chart for the management of acute colonic pseudo-obstruction (ACPO). *CBC,* Complete blood count; *CT,* computed tomography.

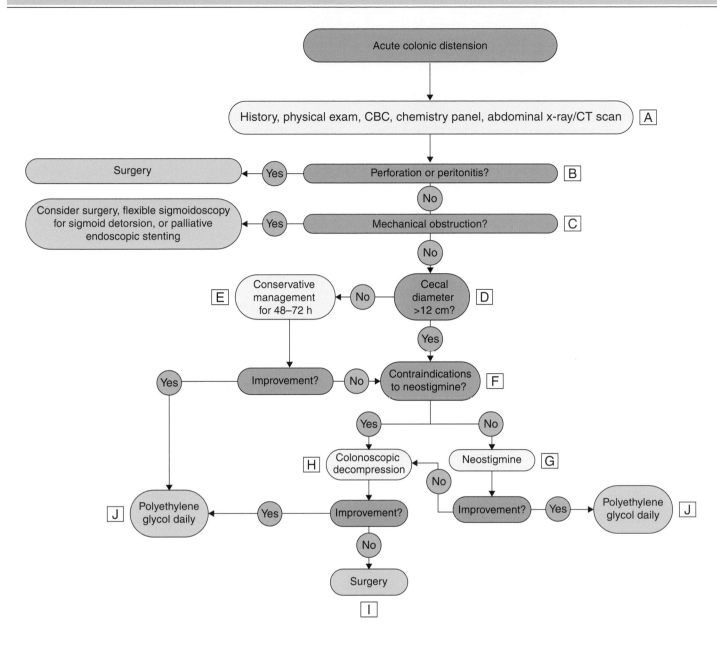

64 | Irritable Bowel Syndrome

Srikrishna Patnana

Irritable bowel syndrome (IBS) is one of the most common gastrointestinal (GI) diseases with a prevalence of approximately 4% using Rome IV criteria.

A. When a patient presents with insidious onset of recurrent abdominal pain in relation to bowel movements, IBS is suspected. Alarm features (GI bleeding, unintentional weight loss, family history of GI cancer or inflammatory bowel disease [IBD] abdominal mass, conjunctival pallor) should be sought out during the clinic encounter. Celiac serologies, C-reactive protein (CRP), and fecal calprotectin should be ordered especially in the presence of diarrhea to evaluate for celiac disease and inflammatory conditions such as IBD.

B. In the presence of alarm symptoms, signs, or abnormal labs, endoscopy and/or cross-sectional imaging need to be performed to exclude microscopic colitis, IBD, and malignancy. If age appropriate, colonoscopy for colon cancer screening should be pursued.

C. In the absence of alarm symptoms, signs, or abnormal labs, a diagnosis of IBS should be made by healthcare providers with confidence. This will reduce delay in initiating appropriate therapy and improve cost-effectiveness of the management. Rome IV criteria for the diagnosis of IBS are: recurrent abdominal pain (at least 1 day/week for the last 3 months with symptom onset 6 months ago) in association with two of the following: pain related to defecation (either increasing or improving pain), associated with a change in stool frequency, or a change in stool form.

D. Carbohydrates are the most common nutrients which trigger IBS symptoms. Fermentable oligosaccharides, disaccharides, monosaccharides, and polyols (FODMAPs) are short-chain carbohydrates, which are poorly digested and absorbed, thereby available for microbial fermentation resulting in GI symptoms. A low FODMAP diet is shown to benefit 60%–70% of patients when properly instituted. Dicyclomine, hyoscyamine, and peppermint oil may be used for treatment of mild abdominal pain in patients with IBS. Neuromodulators, especially tricyclic antidepressants (TCAs), and selective serotonin-norepinephrine reuptake inhibitors (SNRIs) can be used for moderate-severe abdominal pain and global symptoms. Brain-gut behavior therapies should be offered through a GI health psychologist early in the treatment course for the management of IBS symptoms especially in difficult-to-manage cases.

E. For more specific therapies, patients with IBS should be categorized per their predominant abnormal pattern of bowel movements. Patients with constipation-predominant IBS (IBS-C) have hard stools (Bristol stool form scale [BSFS] 1 or 2) >25% of the time, and loose stools (BSFS 6 or 7) <25% of the time. Patients with diarrhea-predominant IBS (IBS-D) have loose stools (BSFS 6 or 7) >25% of the time, and hard stools (BSFS 1 or 2) <25% of the time. Only these two subtypes have specific approved treatments.

F. Polyethylene glycol can be used for mild IBS-C symptoms. If there is no response or in those with moderate-severe symptoms, lubiprostone (8 mcg twice daily), linaclotide (290 mcg once daily), plecanatide (3 mg once daily), or tenapanor (50 mg twice daily) can be used. Improvement in symptoms is seen within 1–2 weeks with linaclotide, and plecanatide, and in approximately 2 months with lubiprostone. Patients who do not respond to 1 or 2 aforementioned treatments or in whom defecatory disorder (DD) is suspected will benefit from evaluation for DD. If such evaluation is positive, patients will benefit from pelvic floor biofeedback therapy.

G. In mild IBS-D patients, loperamide can be tried although data supporting its use are weak. Rifaximin and eluxadoline can be used for more troublesome IBS-D symptoms. Rifaximin is used at a dose of 550 mg thrice daily for 14 days and can be repeated twice for recurrent symptoms. Eluxadoline is used at a dose of 75 mg or 100 mg twice daily. It is contraindicated in patients with alcohol use (>3 drinks/day), history of cholecystectomy, or pancreatitis. In women who do not respond to therapies mentioned earlier, alosetron can be used at dose of 0.5–1 mg twice daily. Its use should be avoided in patients with history of constipation, ischemic colitis, intestinal obstruction/strictures/adhesions/perforation, diverticulitis, or hypercoagulable state.

BIBLIOGRAPHY

1. Lacy BE, Pimentel M, Brenner DM, et al. ACG clinical guideline: management of irritable bowel syndrome. *Am J Gastroenterol.* 2021;116(1):17-44.
2. Chang L, Sultan S, Lembo A, et al. AGA clinical practice guideline on the pharmacological management of irritable bowel syndrome with constipation. *Gastroenterology.* 2022;163(1):118-136.
3. Lembo A, Sultan S, Chang L, et al. AGA clinical practice guideline on the pharmacological management of irritable bowel syndrome with diarrhea. *Gastroenterology.* 2022;163(1):137-151.

ALGORITHM 64.1 Management of irritable bowel syndrome (*IBS*). *CT,* Computed tomography; *DD,* defecatory disorder; *IBS,* irritable bowel syndrome.

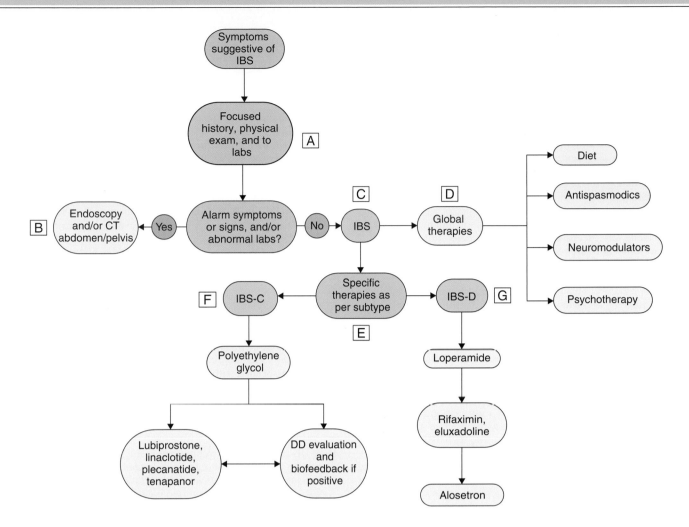

Defecation Disorders

Nikrad Shahnavaz

Defecation disorders are also known as *dyssynergic defecation* (DD) or *outlet obstruction*. The diagnosis of DD requires combination of symptoms of constipation and anorectal tests suggestive of impaired rectal evacuation. These disorders are acquired and may represent learned behavior to avoid pain and discomfort associated with rectal evacuation in patients with severe constipation, active anal fissure, or inflamed hemorrhoids.

A. Symptoms suggestive of DD include hard stools and infrequent defecation along with excessive straining during defecation, use of digital maneuvers to facilitate rectal evacuation, and a sense of anorectal blockage or incomplete evacuation during and after defecation.

B. A digital rectal examination (DRE) should be performed in all patients suspected of having DD. DRE can identify structural abnormalities as well as anal sphincter dysfunction. A DRE should include perianal inspection followed by digital examination to assess stool in the rectum and anal tone at rest and during squeeze and simulated evacuation. Failure of the anal sphincter to relax with simulated defecation or paradoxical contraction suggests DD. The finger is inserted deeper to palpate the puborectalis muscle when the patient is asked to simulate defecation again. Failure of puborectalis muscle to relax also suggests DD. The accuracy of DRE examination in diagnosis of DD has been shown to be comparable with objective studies such as anorectal manometry and balloon expulsion test (BET).

C. Before proceeding with any further tests, management should include optimizing stool consistency with use of water-soluble fiber supplements and laxatives, as well as easing rectal evacuation by using enemas and suppositories. The use of a footstool during defecation and treatment of anal fissure or symptomatic hemorrhoids may help with the management of DD.

D. Anorectal manometry measures rectal sensation and anorectal pressures at rest, during anal sphincter contraction, and simulated defecation. Rectal BET measures the time required to evacuate a balloon filled with 50 mL of warm water in the seated position. These test results should be interpreted together, along with the clinical manifestations, because false-positive and false-negative results are common.

E. Biofeedback therapy includes teaching patients to generate adequate propulsive force and to relax the anal sphincter during evacuation, as well as retraining to enhance rectal sensation and balloon expulsion. Four to six sessions are usually recommended.

F. In patients with inadequate response to biofeedback therapy, barium or magnetic resonance (MR) defecography studies are indicated to confirm DD and to rule out structural abnormalities such as solitary rectal ulcers, rectoceles, and rectal prolapse. Barium defecography is performed in the seated position, while MR defecography is performed in the supine position and provides better assessments of pelvic organ prolapse and pelvic floor motion.

G. Structural abnormalities of the pelvic floor can be found in asymptomatic individuals and do not require surgical correction. Similarly, surgical repair of structural abnormalities in patients with evacuation difficulty does not usually result in resolution of symptoms and is not recommended in most cases. Exceptions include overt rectal prolapse, a large (>5 cm), nonemptying rectocele and when rectocele is associated with gynecological symptoms such as bulging in the perineum or protrusion through the vaginal introitus. When sigmoidoceles and enteroceles are symptomatic, they may be treated with surgical repair (sacrocolpopexy) after careful radiological evaluation.

H. If DD is ruled out with physiologic studies and defecography, slow transit constipation should be suspected and confirmed with radiopaque marker study or wireless motility capsule. In severe disabling cases unresponsive to optimized laxative therapy, subtotal colectomy with ileorectal anastomosis could be considered.

BIBLIOGRAPHY

1. Iturrino JC, Lembo AJ. Constipation Sleisenger and Fordtran's Gastrointestinal and Liver Disease, 11th edition, Elsevier; 2020.
2. Wald A, Bharucha AE, Limketkai B, et al. ACG clinical guidelines: management of benign anorectal disorders. *Am J Gastroenterol.* 2021;116(10):1987-2008.

ALGORITHM 65.1 Evaluation and management of dyssynergic defecation (DD) *MR,* Magnetic resonance.

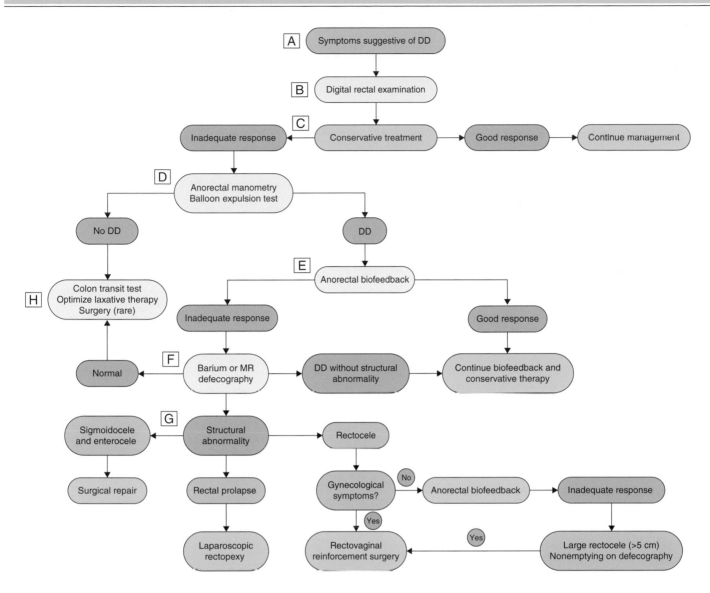

66 Acute Severe Ulcerative Colitis

Manjusha Das

Ulcerative colitis (UC) is a chronic inflammatory bowel disease with peak onset in early adulthood. The diagnosis should be suspected in patients with hematochezia, urgency, and tenesmus. The disease follows a relapsing and remitting pattern. Any patient with a diagnosis of UC and acute worsening of symptoms should undergo early evaluation and treatment.

A. Acute severe UC is defined as the presence of six or more bowel movements per day associated with signs of systemic toxicity (tachycardia, fever, anemia, or elevated erythrocyte sedimentation rate [ESR]). Other symptoms to assess the disease severity are urgency, abdominal pain, and weight loss.

B. Acute severe UC requires inpatient hospital admission for urgent evaluation and treatment. Abdominal examination should evaluate for signs of surgical abdomen, including guarding, rigidity, and rebound tenderness. Laboratory workup includes complete blood count (CBC), comprehensive metabolic panel (CMP), ESR, and C-reactive protein (CRP). It is imperative to rule out concomitant superimposed infections. If *Clostridioides difficile* is present, it is imperative to start treatment with vancomycin immediately regardless of ongoing treatment for UC. Patients should receive intravenous (IV) fluid and deep vein thrombosis (DVT) prophylaxis. Radiographic imaging with either abdominal x-ray or computed tomography (CT) is performed to rule out megacolon or perforation. Flexible sigmoidoscopy with biopsy is performed to confirm the diagnosis and rule out *Cytomegalovirus* colitis.

C. Patients who are found to have acute severe UC with complications such as toxic megacolon, perforation, and severe refractory hematochezia due to fulminant colitis should undergo surgery and colectomy.

D. The first-line treatment of acute severe UC is IV steroids with methylprednisolone at 60 mg per day to induce remission.

E. Patients who respond to IV steroids can transition to oral prednisone. A response to IV steroids is observed with improvements in any or all clinical symptoms including urgency, frequency of bowel movements, and hematochezia. Dosing for oral prednisone is 40 mg daily. Patients are generally discharged with close outpatient follow-up to initiate maintenance therapy with biologics or Janus kinase (JAK) inhibitors.

F. In patients who do not respond to IV steroids within 48–72 hours, rescue therapy is given with either infliximab or cyclosporine. Randomized clinical trials have shown that infliximab and cyclosporine are similarly effective as rescue therapy in acute severe UC. The choice between infliximab and cyclosporine should be decided based on the patient's prior exposure to immunomodulator and anti-tumor necrosis factor (TNF) therapy, albumin level, and local expertise. Infliximab and cyclosporine do not increase postoperative complications of colectomy and surgery should not be deferred based on the exposure to these agents. Small case series suggest that tofacitinib might be effective in inducing remission in patients with acute severe UC who have previously received biologic therapy.

G. In patients who respond to rescue therapy with infliximab, dosing is repeated at 2 and 6 weeks, and then every 8 weeks. Patients who respond to IV cyclosporin should be transitioned to oral cyclosporin and thiopurine. Vedolizumab is an alternative to thiopurine to maintain remission.

H. Patients who do not respond to IV infliximab or cyclosporin within 3–5 days, should undergo surgery with proctocolectomy. Patients who do not respond to initial infliximab dose of 5 mg/kg may be given the second infusion of infliximab at a dose of 10 mg/kg before considering surgery.

BIBLIOGRAPHY

1. Rubin DT, Ananthakrishnan AN, Siegel CA, Sauer BG, Long MD. ACG clinical guideline: ulcerative colitis in adults. *Am J Gastroenterol.* 2019;114(3): 384-413.
2. Laharie D, Bourreille A, Branche J, et al. Ciclosporin versus infliximab in patients with severe ulcerative colitis refractory to intravenous steroids: a parallel, open-label randomised controlled trial. *Lancet.* 2012;380(9857): 1909-1915. https://doi:10.1016/S0140-6736(12)61084-8.
3. Williams JG, Alam MF, Alrubaiy L, et al. Infliximab versus ciclosporin for steroid-resistant acute severe ulcerative colitis (CONSTRUCT): a mixed methods, open-label, pragmatic randomised trial. *Lancet Gastroenterol Hepatol.* 2016;1(1):15-24.

ALGORITHM 66.1 Flowchart for the workup and management of a patient with acute severe ulcerative colitis. *CBC,* Complete blood count; *CMP,* comprehensive metabolic panel; *CRP,* C-reactive protein; *CT,* computed tomography; *DVT,* deep vein thrombosis; *ESR,* erythrocyte sedimentation rate; *HBV,* hepatitis B virus; *IV,* intravenous; *JAK,* Janus kinase; *NPO,* nil per os; *PPD,* purified protein derivative.

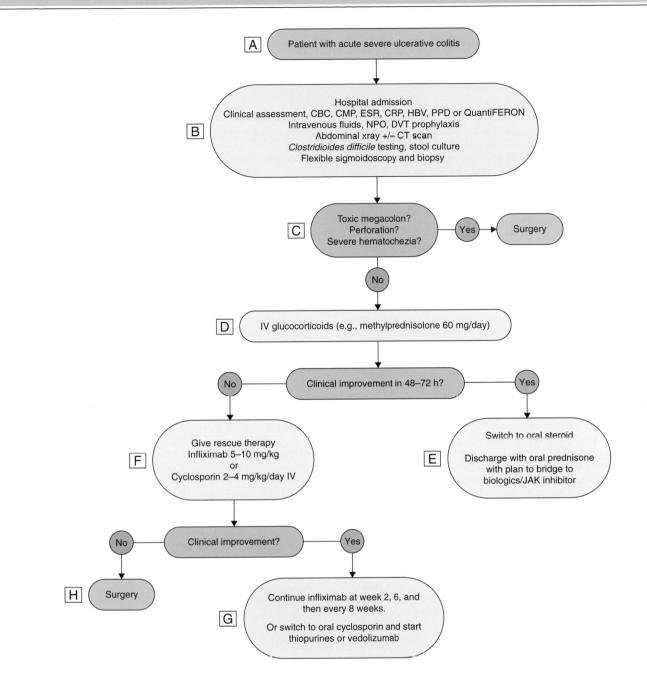

67 Treatment of Ulcerative Colitis

Mohammed Razvi

Ulcerative colitis is an autoimmune inflammatory condition affecting the mucosal lining of the colon. Colonic inflammation can initially affect the rectum alone, but disease could progress to cause proctosigmoiditis or even pancolitis. In severe or refractory cases, patients can experience significant morbidity, which could even lead to colectomy. Medical therapy using a variety of medications, such as biologic therapy and small molecule agents, has led to improvements in long-term disease control and has decreased incidence of complications such as colectomy or colorectal cancer.

A. The first step in management of the ulcerative colitis patient is to assess the extent and severity of disease, as this information has implications for subsequent treatment steps. Extent of disease is best determined with colonoscopy examination, which can assess if inflammation involves rectum alone, both rectum and left colon up to the splenic flexure, or both distal and proximal colon beyond the splenic flexure. The areas of involvement are important particularly for mild to moderate disease severity as topical therapies are chosen based on the areas affected by inflammation. In addition, the disease severity at presentation helps to determine if 5-aminosalicylic acid (5-ASA) therapy can serve as the initial treatment choice such as for mild-moderate disease or if biologic therapy and immunomodulator therapy are needed as the first step in therapy such as for moderate-severe disease. There are several severity scales commonly used in clinical practice, but the Mayo score is a prevalent severity index widely used today in clinical trials and routine practice. The Mayo score incorporates factors such as stool frequency, extent of rectal bleeding, mucosal appearance at endoscopy, and global disease activity rating by a physician to calculate severity of disease. Other clinical indicators can also help in assessment of severity including inflammatory markers, presence of anemia or iron deficiency, and extraintestinal manifestations, among others.

B. Though topical therapies such as mesalamine suppositories and enemas are effective management options for proctitis and left-sided disease, patients may be averse to the mode of administration or may face financial barriers with these therapies. Thus, oral 5-ASA may be the initial choice of therapy in these patients if compliance to medication is more optimal with this formulation. Regardless of which 5-ASA formulation is chosen as the initial therapy, if disease remains uncontrolled despite administration, then oral therapy can be added to topical therapy, or vice versa, depending on which type of therapy was started initially. Similarly, oral 5-ASA is generally started at standard dose with the option to increase to high dose if disease remains uncontrolled.

C. In cases where 5-ASA is not sufficient to induce remission, steroid therapy may be required for initial disease control. Steroid therapy can include topical rectal administration such as with suppository, enema, or foam-based products for proctitis or left-sided disease. For pancolitis, oral steroid administration such as with prednisone or budesonide may be required. The goal of steroid therapy is to provide the shortest duration needed while other therapies take effect followed by discontinuation. If steroids are unable to be discontinued or several courses are required, then consideration of biologic therapy and immunomodulators will be needed.

D. In ulcerative colitis patients with moderate to severe disease being treated in the outpatient setting, the initial therapy choice can be either vedolizumab or an antitumor necrosis factor (anti-TNF) agent (with or without immunomodulator therapy). Vedolizumab is an attractive first-line agent due to its favorable side-effect profile and minimal immunosuppression. Studies have shown that vedolizumab works best in anti-TNF naïve patients, providing further evidence that vedolizumab should be considered before any other biologic agent. The VARSITY trial, the first head-to-head trial comparing medical therapies for ulcerative colitis, found that vedolizumab was superior to adalimumab in achieving clinical remission and endoscopic improvement. Despite this, adalimumab remains a potential first-line therapy for ulcerative colitis along with other anti-TNF therapies such as infliximab or golimumab, though many experts recommend infliximab as the most effective anti-TNF therapy for this condition. Studies have suggested that anti-TNF therapy is less effective after failing a second anti-TNF agent; thus it is better to switch to alternate biologic therapy after the second anti-TNF agent rather than continuing to a third agent in the same therapy class. In fact, experts now routinely recommend that in ulcerative colitis patients who have previously been exposed to infliximab, consideration of ustekinumab or Janus tyrosine kinase (JAK) inhibitor therapy as next steps in treatment should be made over using vedolizumab or adalimumab in this clinical scenario. Immunomodulator therapy given in combination with anti-TNF therapy is shown to be more effective particularly in prevention of drug antibody formation, but with the potential increased risk of side effects and further immunosuppression. However, anti-TNF monotherapy is still effective and safe; thus it can be used as the initial therapy choice, with subsequent addition of immunomodulator for combination therapy if low-level antibodies develop or if switching to a second anti-TNF agent is due to failure of the first agent. Inadequate initial response or loss of response to therapies such as anti-TNF therapy, vedolizumab, or ustekinumab should result in reactive assessment of drug trough levels. Dose escalation, in which the dosage or frequency of therapy is increased, should be pursued to raise levels or drive down antibodies to recapture therapy response. Refer to Chapter 71 (Biologic Therapy in Inflammatory Bowel Disease) for further discussion of this topic. Following trials of vedolizumab and anti-TNF therapy, the next step is to transition to ustekinumab and small molecule therapies. Ustekinumab has been shown to remain effective following anti-TNF exposure, which allows this medication to serve as an excellent second-line option. JAK inhibitors, such as tofacitinib and upadacitinib, are considered potent therapies with ease of administration via oral route, but can have significant immunosuppressive effects, which can increase the risk of infectious complications. Ozanimod is also recently available as a small molecule therapy for ulcerative colitis, but its position within treatment algorithms has yet to be established.

E. The severe ulcerative colitis patient requiring inpatient hospital admission due to fulminant disease will initially require intravenous (IV) steroids to attempt induction of remission. This is discussed in detail in Chapter 66 (Acute Severe Ulcerative Colitis), and is summarized below. Response to IV steroids should be evaluated daily with objective criteria such as trending serum inflammatory markers and monitoring of stool output, along with subjective criteria such as

---

ALGORITHM 67.1 Flowchart for the treatment of ulcerative colitis. *5-ASA*, 5-Aminosalicylic acid; *anti-TNF*, antitumor necrosis factor; *IMM*, immunomodulator; *IV*, intravenous; *JAK*, Janus tyrosine kinase.

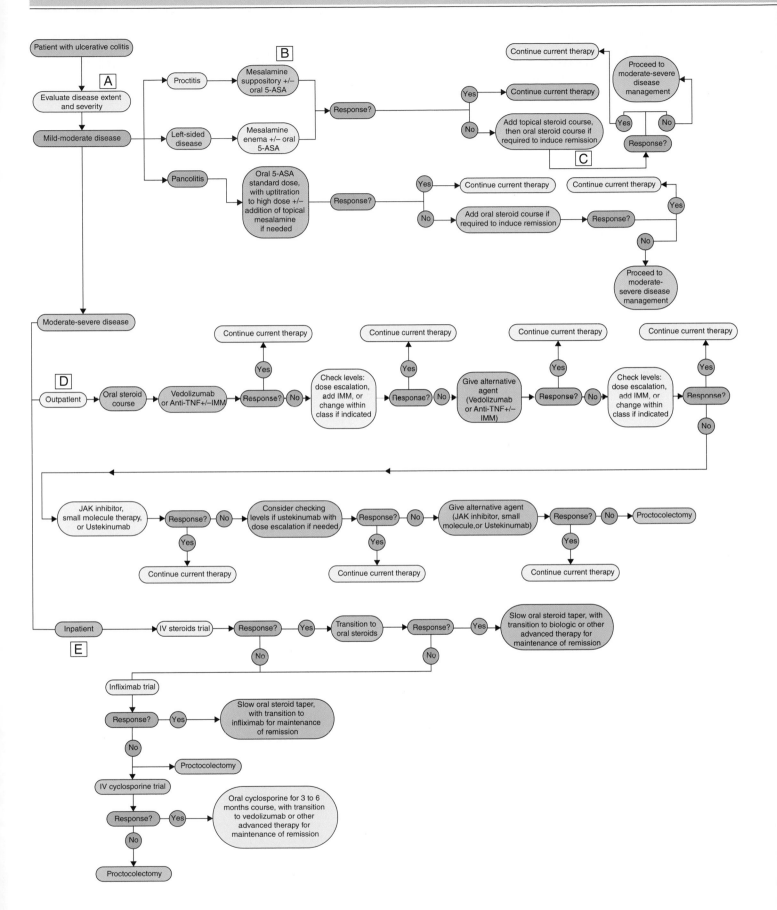

amount of blood in the stool and consistency of the stool. Response to steroids may take up to 72 hours or more. If response to IV steroids is achieved, then transition to oral steroids with additional 24–48 hours of monitoring is needed to ensure that the patient does not relapse while taking oral therapy. Of note, if the patient is infliximab naïve, then this can be started during the hospitalization while receiving concomitant steroid therapy; otherwise, initiation of infliximab can be deferred to the outpatient setting if there is adequate response to steroid therapy. Unfortunately, many patients with fulminant colitis requiring hospitalization have already tried and failed infliximab, though if there is doubt as to whether the patient was challenged with optimized dose escalation in the past, then infliximab may still be an option. Cyclosporine salvage therapy is an option when infliximab has been previously tried and failed by the patient or if infliximab therapy did not induce remission; however, cyclosporine use is limited by adverse effects and is recommended for otherwise healthy patients being treated in centers with significant experience using the protocol. Due to concern for significant immunosuppression, cyclosporine is generally used as bridge therapy to vedolizumab, and long-term monotherapy should be avoided. Ultimately, if medical therapy fails, then surgical therapy with proctocolectomy remains an option. Early evaluation by colorectal surgery colleagues is recommended in case emergent colectomy is required due to complications or failure of medical therapy.

BIBLIOGRAPHY

1. Dassopoulos T, Cohen RD, Scherl EJ, et al. Ulcerative colitis care pathway. *Gastroenterology*. 2015;149:238-245.
2. Feuerstein JD, Isaacs KL, Schneider Y, et al. AGA clinical practice guidelines on the management of moderate to severe ulcerative colitis. *Gastroenterology*. 2020;158:1450-1461.
3. Ko CW, Singh S, Feuerstein JD, et al. AGA clinical practice guidelines on the management of mild-to-moderate ulcerative colitis. *Gastroenterology*. 2019;156:748-764.
4. Rubin DT, Ananthakrishnan AN, Siegel CA, et al. ACG clinical guideline: ulcerative colitis in adults. *Am J Gastroenterol*. 2019;114:384-413.

68 Crohn's Disease

Jasna I. Beard

Crohn's disease (CD) is a clinically diagnosed multisystemic idiopathic inflammatory disease. While it can lead to a variety of constitutional, rheumatologic, dermatologic, and other symptoms, the predominant manifestation is gastrointestinal (GI). Commonly, it presents as weight loss, failure to thrive, abdominal pain, diarrhea, and GI bleeding. Its course can be complicated by immunosuppression and associated infections, GI perforation or abscess formation, or extraintestinal manifestations (EIMs) such as eye or joint disease. Conversely, the disease itself as well as its treatment (e.g., steroids) can complicate comorbid conditions like diabetes, heart disease, or chronic infections. The vast majority of patients do not experience extension of GI disease involvement beyond what is present at time of diagnosis, though some can. For example, a patient with terminal ileitis can develop extraintestinal Crohn manifestations over the years, but generally does not experience extension of the GI disease beyond the ileum.

Treatment of CD is generally approached with a multidisciplinary team of radiologists, surgeons, pathologists, and gastroenterologists. The team evolves based on the patient's manifestations to include other subspecialties, as needed. The focus of treatment is primarily on suppression of inflammation with the use of agents like steroids, tumor necrosis factor-alpha (TNFα) inhibitors, and immunomodulators (IMMs). The choice of treatment hinges on the disease severity, extent, phenotype, and patient comorbidities.

A. The first step after diagnosis is to define the disease severity and patient features. Mild CD is generally defined as GI inflammation in an ambulatory patient who retains GI function (i.e., tolerates oral intake, has less than 10% weight loss, and has symptoms that do not significantly impact quality of life). All other patients are defined as moderate-to-severe CD.

B. Patient demographics and comorbidities can impact the disease evolution as well as choice of treatment. For example, young age at diagnosis makes severe disease more likely; reproductive plans or presence of cardiovascular disease can narrow the choice of treatment.

C. CD extent of involvement at time of diagnosis often informs choice of treatment. Inflammation can affect any segment of the GI tract and is defined as gastroduodenal, small bowel, colonic, perianal, or a combination. Furthermore, extraintestinal CD can include ocular, skin, or joint disease, for example.

D. When categorizing the GI tract manifestations, it is important to define the CD phenotype as inflammatory, stricturing (also called *fibrostenosing*), or penetrating (also called *fistulizing*). Mild disease tends to remain inflammatory-only, while more severe involvement can include fistula or abscess formation.

E. Lastly, when approaching a patient with a CD diagnosis, it is very important to determine if the disease is currently active or "flaring." Since there are no pathognomonic features of CD, this is done by a combination of the clinical assessment, radiologic features, and serologic inflammatory markers. For example, a patient may present with new diarrhea, abdominal pain, enhancing thickened bowel wall on cross-sectional imaging, and laboratory tests showing anemia and an elevated fecal calprotectin level. While the majority of patients will experience intermittent disease flares, a small proportion may have

disease that remains quiescent for many years. Those with quiescent disease generally also require treatment to prevent future flares, if treatment is consistent with the patient's goals.

F. When evaluating a symptomatic CD patient, the first step is to determine if the symptoms are primarily due to active CD or due to other contributors. This requires consideration of bile acid diarrhea (commonly seen with ileal disease or resection), small intestinal bacterial overgrowth (commonly seen with stricturing CD), medication side effects, and infection, among others. Possible infectious agents range from common community-acquired (e.g., viral gastroenteritis) or rarer ones seen in immunosuppressed patients (e.g., cytomegalovirus).

G. If the evaluation determines that symptoms are due to acute flare of CD, treatment generally starts with a steroid taper administered orally or intravenously, based on symptom severity.

H. While the steroid taper can quickly control symptoms and induce remission of active disease, steroids are not recommended for use in the maintenance of remission. It is important to use shared decision-making with the patient and consider the features discussed earlier (e.g., disease severity, phenotype, extent, and patient factors) in determining a strategy for maintenance of remission. Mild inflammatory ileocolonic CD can remain under control with use of budesonide (ileal- or colonic-release, dependent on disease location). Patients with mild CD but comorbidities that place them at high risk for complications in setting of a flare or those with moderate-to-severe CD should consider combination therapy of IMMs and biologic agents, with preference for infliximab, if no contraindications exist.

I. It is of paramount importance to verify efficacy of treatment when it comes to CD, as untreated persistent inflammation increases risk of recurrent severe activity, colorectal cancer, and comorbidities such as malnutrition and anemia. This is generally done by a clinical, radiographic, and histologic reassessment approximately 6 months after new medication or a change in therapy.

J. If the patient is determined to have reached clinical and histologic remission upon reassessment, it is appropriate to monitor for disease recurrence. Clinical follow-up also includes assessment for side effects and health maintenance measures, such as bone density scans, immunization, cancer prevention, and nutritional evaluations.

K. It is important to always thoroughly assess CD for presence of complications, such as obstruction or perforation that require surgical intervention to induce disease remission. While practices vary by institution and perioperative management of CD deserves a dedicated review, if the disease flare is deemed to have occurred despite adequate medical therapy, patients generally require a postoperative medication change to maintain remission. Refer to Chapter 70—Postoperative Management of Crohn's Disease for further discussion on this topic.

L. Patients with active CD who do not require surgical intervention can consider medical management by either "step-up" therapy

---

ALGORITHM 68.1 Management of Crohn's disease (CD). *EIM*, extraintestinal manifestation; *IMM*, immunomodulator; *IV*, intravenous; *PO*, per mouth; *SIBO*, small intestinal bacterial overgrowth; *TDM*, therapeutic drug monitoring; *TGN*, thioguanine; *TNFα*, tumor necrosis factor-alpha.

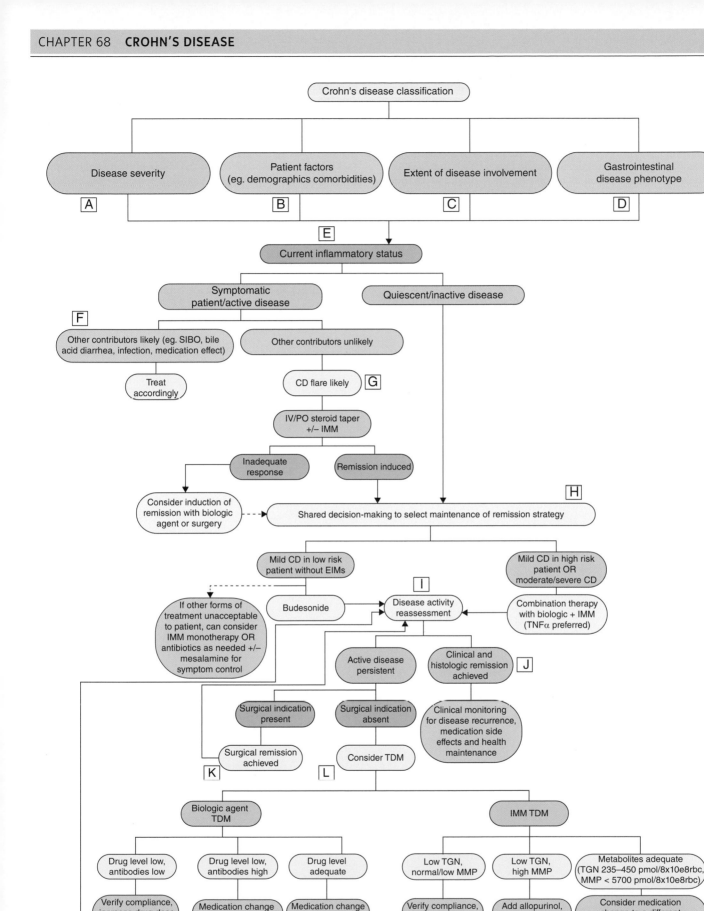

from budesonide to a biologic agent or therapeutic drug monitoring (TDM), where applicable. TDM of biologic agents can inform the next steps by determining the serum medication level and the presence of antibodies to the medication. Antibodies inactivate the medication, without causing patient symptoms themselves. The goal medication level varies and is specific to each agent. If a medication level is below goal and no antibodies are present, one can consider verifying compliance and increasing the medication dose or frequency. If the medication level is low due to high titer of antibodies, one can consider a change to an agent within the same class. However, if the medication level is adequate and no antibodies present, yet the disease recurs, the patient is considered nonresponsive to that agent and a switch to an agent of a *different* class is considered. In general, TNFα agents are the first-line choice, followed by ustekinumab and vedolizumab, favored over certolizumab. If the disease phenotype includes abscesses or fistulas, it is advisable to add antibiotics at induction alongside biologic agents. Refer to Chapter 71— Biologic Therapy in Inflammatory Bowel Disease for further discussion of management of nonresponse or loss of response to biologic therapy. While IMMs are preferred in conjunction with TNFα agents, their role is less clear with biologic agents of other classes. Lastly, TDM can be used to optimize efficacy and minimize toxicity of IMMs, similar to its role in managing biologic agents, by measuring the levels of thioguanine (TGN) and methylmercaptopurine (MMP). The disease monitoring cycle would then restart with the new medication regimen and include a 6-month reassessment of response.

BIBLIOGRAPHY

1. Feuerstein JD, Ho EY, Shmidt E, et al. AGA clinical practice guidelines on the medical management of moderate to severe luminal and perianal fistulizing Crohn's disease. *Gastroenterology*. 2021;160(7):2496-2508.
2. Lichtenstein GR, Loftus EV, Isaacs KL, et al. ACG clinical guideline: management of Crohn's disease in adults. *Am J Gastroenterol*. 2018;113(4):481-517.

69 Management of Crohn's Disease in Pregnancy

Mohammed Razvi

Crohn's disease is an autoimmune inflammatory condition that affects the gastrointestinal system and can result in significant morbidity, quality of life issues, and complex clinical scenarios. Many Crohn's disease patients are women of reproductive age. Thus, it is imperative to consider the treatment of Crohn's disease during pregnancy since maternal health, fetal growth, and the labor and delivery process can all be affected by this important disease and its subsequent management.

A. The management of the pregnant Crohn's disease patient requires a multidisciplinary approach from a variety of experts. These patients are best served by involvement of a gastroenterologist who specializes in inflammatory bowel disease and a maternal-fetal medicine specialist. The patient may benefit from other providers such as a colorectal surgeon, clinical nutritionist, or lactation consultant.

B. The first decision point in the initial evaluation and management of Crohn's disease in the setting of pregnancy is to assess the disease activity at the beginning of gestation. The best predictor of a healthy and successful pregnancy and delivery for both the mother and infant in Crohn's disease patients is the achievement and maintenance of remission of disease. Ideally, the patient is already in remission, confirmed by routine clinical, biochemical, and endoscopic evaluations, and on stable maintenance therapy before conception; thus therapy can be continued with the required additional monitoring and evaluation during the pregnancy. However, depending on the individual clinical scenario, there will be patients who did not receive routine care before conception, or those who may start flaring during pregnancy, and thus management of active disease may be required during the pregnancy.

C. There is no evidence to suggest that vaginal delivery increases the risk of development of Crohn's disease in the fetus. Thus, most Crohn's disease patients can safely proceed with vaginal delivery. However, if there is a history of rectovaginal fistula, then vaginal delivery should be avoided to prevent recurrence or other complications of the prior fistula site that may occur from trauma of the rectovaginal wall during delivery. Similar complications can occur if vaginal delivery occurs with active perianal disease, so these patients are best suited to proceed with cesarean delivery. A detailed perineal examination near full-term gestation is important to guide the labor and delivery

process. Of note, pharmacological prophylaxis for venous thromboembolic disease is generally recommended following delivery in patients with active Crohn's disease flare and patients who undergo cesarean delivery.

D. Regarding medical therapy in pregnant Crohn's disease patients who achieved remission, continuation of current biologic therapy is important to maintain disease control. All biologic therapies used for Crohn's disease management are considered safe to use in pregnancy for both mother and fetus. Certolizumab pegol has the added benefit of not crossing the placental barrier; thus some biologic naïve patients may opt to begin this agent during pregnancy to control active disease depending on their goals and preferences. However, switching from an alternate biologic therapy on which the patient's disease is already controlled to certolizumab pegol may confer the risk of the disease becoming uncontrolled during pregnancy, if there is inadequate response to certolizumab pegol. In addition, though thiopurines are considered safe to use in pregnancy, due to potential increased infection risk to the infant, patients who use combination therapy with biologic and thiopurine may decide to withdraw the thiopurine during pregnancy.

E. Due to potential complications and side effects of thiopurines, which could negatively affect pregnant patients, such as leukopenia, photosensitivity, or pancreatitis, it is recommended that pregnant patients are not given thiopurines as a new-start medication. Methotrexate is considered a teratogen and should not be used in pregnant patients or women of childbearing age who may become pregnant. Endoscopy or other procedures should be considered only if there is a strong indication that could change the management or course of the disease.

BIBLIOGRAPHY

1. Lichtenstein GR, Loftus EV, Isaacs KL, et al. ACG clinical guideline: management of Crohn's disease in adults. *Am J Gastroenterol.* 2018;113:481-517.
2. Mahadevan U, Robinson C, Bernasko N, et al. Inflammatory bowel disease in pregnancy clinical care pathway: a report from the American Gastroenterological Association IBD Parenthood Project Working Group. *Gastroenterology.* 2019;156:1508-1524.
3. Selinger CP, Nelson-Piercy C, Fraser A, et al. IBD in pregnancy: recent advances, practical management. *Frontline Gastroenterol.* 2021;12:214-224.

ALGORITHM 69.1 Flow chart for the management of Crohn's disease in pregnancy. *BPP,* Biophysical profile; *CBC,* complete blood count; *CRP,* C-reactive protein; *LFT,* liver function test; *MRI,* magnetic resonance imaging; *NST,* nonstress test.

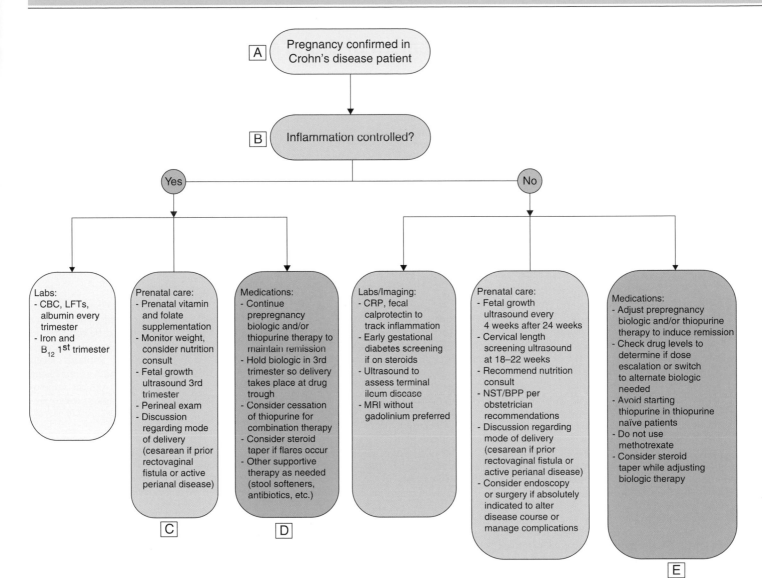

A Pregnancy confirmed in Crohn's disease patient

B Inflammation controlled?

Yes

No

Labs:
- CBC, LFTs, albumin every trimester
- Iron and B$_{12}$ 1st trimester

C Prenatal care:
- Prenatal vitamin and folate supplementation
- Monitor weight, consider nutrition consult
- Fetal growth ultrasound 3rd trimester
- Perineal exam
- Discussion regarding mode of delivery (cesarean if prior rectovaginal fistula or active perianal disease)

D Medications:
- Continue prepregnancy biologic and/or thiopurine therapy to maintain remission
- Hold biologic in 3rd trimester so delivery takes place at drug trough
- Consider cessation of thiopurine for combination therapy
- Consider steroid taper if flares occur
- Other supportive therapy as needed (stool softeners, antibiotics, etc.)

Labs/Imaging:
- CRP, fecal calprotectin to track inflammation
- Early gestational diabetes screening if on steroids
- Ultrasound to assess terminal ileum disease
- MRI without gadolinium preferred

Prenatal care:
- Fetal growth ultrasound every 4 weeks after 24 weeks
- Cervical length screening ultrasound at 18–22 weeks
- Recommend nutrition consult
- NST/BPP per obstetrician recommendations
- Discussion regarding mode of delivery (cesarean if prior rectovaginal fistula or active perianal disease)
- Consider endoscopy or surgery if absolutely indicated to alter disease course or manage complications

E Medications:
- Adjust prepregnancy biologic and/or thiopurine therapy to induce remission
- Check drug levels to determine if dose escalation or switch to alternate biologic needed
- Avoid starting thiopurine in thiopurine naïve patients
- Do not use methotrexate
- Consider steroid taper while adjusting biologic therapy

70 Postoperative Management of Crohn's Disease

Manjusha Das

The most common surgical resection in Crohn's disease is an ileocolonic resection and primary anastomosis due to refractory disease in the ileocolonic bowel segment. Studies suggest that an end-to-end anastomosis leads to better quality of life and less healthcare utilization compared with side-to-side anastomosis. Patients who undergo surgical resection have disease recurrence most commonly at the site of the surgical anastomosis. Without medical prophylaxis, endoscopic recurrence develops in approximately 70% of patients 1-year postresection. The 5-year cumulative risk of clinical recurrence is 40%–50%. Several medications were shown to decrease the risk of postoperative recurrence of Crohn's disease, such as thiopurines, metronidazole, and anti-tumor necrosis factor (TNF) therapy. The strongest data support the use of the anti-TNF agent infliximab.

A. Once the patient undergoes ileocolonic resection, the decision to give postoperative prophylaxis depends on the presence of risk factors for recurrent Crohn's disease. Patient-related factors include cigarette smoking, young age at the time of surgery (<30 years), and young age of onset of disease. Disease-related factors include shorter duration of disease before surgery, more than one resection, long (>10 cm) segment disease, and penetrating or fistulizing complications. There are no specific guidelines to risk stratify those risk factors. However, those considered high risk are patients who smoke, those with fistulizing disease, or those with two or more prior surgeries. Those with moderate risk have risk factors other than those associated with high risk. Patients are considered low risk for recurrent disease if they have a long-standing Crohn's disease undergoing the first surgery, with mild inflammatory or fibrostenotic disease involving a short bowel segment.

B. Postoperatively, all patients who are smokers should be strongly advised to quit smoking to prevent recurrent disease. Mesalamine is of limited benefit in preventing postoperative Crohn's disease. Nitroimidazole antibiotics (e.g., metronidazole) at doses between 1 and 2 g/day can be used after ileocolonic resection to prevent recurrence. In patients who are at high risk for recurrent disease, anti-TNF therapy is recommended within 4 weeks of surgery. Adding thiopurine to anti-TNF therapy reduces immunogenicity and decreases loss of response. In patients with moderate risk factors for recurrent disease, monotherapy with an immunomodulator is appropriate. No prophylactic therapy is necessary in patients classified as low risk.

C. Colonoscopy is performed at 6 months postoperatively to examine for recurrent disease at the neoterminal ileum and anastomosis. Postoperative disease recurrence is scored by the Rutgeerts endoscopic recurrence score.

D. A normal examination (no inflammation) is graded as 0, and a score of 1 indicates five or fewer aphthous lesions. These patients are considered to have endoscopic remission with low risk of disease progression. There is no need to adjust therapy, and repeat colonoscopy is performed at 1- to 3-year intervals.

E. Patients with a score of i2, i3, or i4 are considered to have endoscopic recurrence. Corticosteroids should be considered to help induce remission in symptomatic patients. Therapy should be escalated to anti-TNF with or without thiopurine. If the patient is already on anti-TNF therapy, then drug trough levels and antibody levels should be obtained to guide further management such as increasing the drug dose or frequency or switching to a drug from the same or different class (refer to Chapter 71—Biologic Therapy in Inflammatory Bowel Disease).

BIBLIOGRAPHY

1. Nguyen GC, Loftus EV Jr., Hirano I, et al. American Gastroenterological Association Institute guideline on the management of Crohn's disease after surgical resection. *Gastroenterology.* 2017;152:(1)271-275. https://doi.org/10.1053/j.gastro.2016.10.038.
2. Regueiro M, Feagan BG, Zou B, et al. Infliximab reduces endoscopic, but not clinical, recurrence of Crohn's disease after ileocolonic resection. *Gastroenterology.* 2016;150:(7)1568-1578. https://doi.org/10.1053/j.gastro.2016.02.072.
3. Gajendran M, Bauer AJ, Bauer BM, et al. Ileocecal anastomosis type significantly influences long-term functional status, quality of life, and healthcare utilization in postoperative Crohn's disease patients independent of inflammation recurrence. *Am J Gastroenterol.* 2018;113:(4)576-583. https://doi.org/10.1038/ajg.2018.13.
4. De Cruz P, Kamm MA, Hamilton AL, et al. Crohn's disease management after intestinal resection: a randomised trial. *Lancet.* 2015;385:(9976)1406-1417. https://doi.org/10.1016/S0140-6736(14)61908-5.

ALGORITHM 70.1 Flowchart for the workup and management of postoperative Crohn's disease. *TNF,* Tumor necrosis factor.

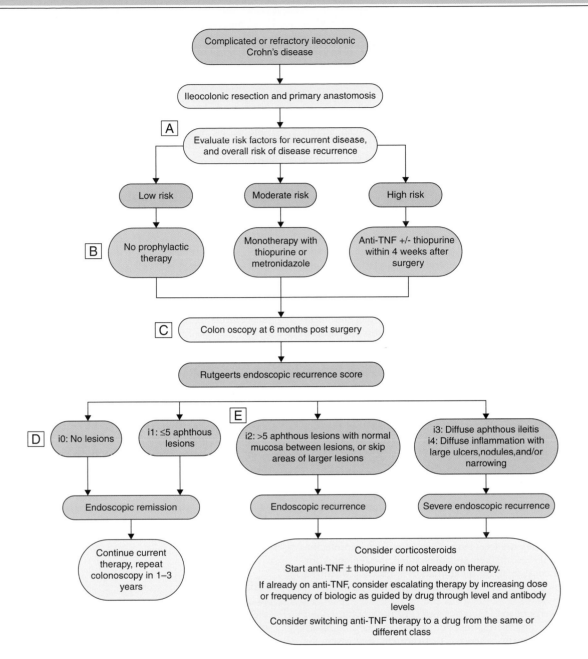

71 | Biologic Therapy in Inflammatory Bowel Disease

Emad Qayed

Biologic therapy for inflammatory bowel disease (IBD) includes anti-tumor necrosis agents (infliximab, adalimumab, certolizumab, golimumab), antiintegrins (vedolizumab), and antiinterleukin (ustekinumab). Recently, oral drugs have been approved for the treatment of ulcerative colitis: Janus kinase (JAK) inhibitors (tofacitinib and upadacitinib) and sphingosine-1-phosphate (S1P) receptor modulators (ozanimod). These drugs are classified as "small molecules" and are usually given as a second-line treatment for ulcerative colitis. This algorithm covers the overall approach to starting biologic therapy for IBD, and management of nonresponse or loss of response. The choice of the initial and subsequent biologic therapy depends on several factors, including the patient's age, comorbid conditions, presence of extraintestinal manifestations, cost, and coverage of the drug by medical insurance.

A. Before starting biologic therapy for IBD, the diagnosis should be confirmed by reviewing the clinical history, endoscopic, and histologic findings. Testing for latent tuberculosis and chronic hepatitis B is required before starting biologic therapy.

B. If the patient does not respond to initial induction biologic therapy, then adherence to therapy should be confirmed. Consider repeating the endoscopy to confirm presence of active inflammation. If adherence is confirmed and active inflammation is present, then this is classified as "primary nonresponse." Switching to another biologic with a different mechanism of action (MOA) is appropriate. In ulcerative colitis, switching to a small molecule is reasonable.

C. If the patient responds to initial induction biologic therapy, then maintenance therapy should be continued. If the patient achieves stable clinical remission, the drug should be continued, and colonoscopy should be performed to confirm endoscopic remission. An alternative approach in ulcerative colitis patients who are in clinical remission is to measure fecal biomarkers (e.g., fecal calprotectin, fecal lactoferrin). If these markers are not elevated, then colonoscopy can be deferred because active inflammation is unlikely when the patient is in clinical remission and fecal biomarkers are normal.

D. If a patient who responded to therapy has recurrent symptoms, then this is considered "loss of response" or "secondary nonresponse." In these patients, confirm adherence to treatment, and assess for the presence of active inflammation using laboratory markers (erythrocyte sedimentation rate [ESR], C-reactive protein [CRP], fecal calprotectin), endoscopy, and/or imaging.

E. Patients with intraabdominal abscess, intractable fistulas, toxic megacolon, fulminant colitis, and refractory hemorrhage should undergo surgical therapy.

F. Patients with short and well-defined strictures may benefit from endoscopic therapy (e.g., endoscopic balloon dilation). More complex fibrostenotic disease requires surgery.

G. Patients without active inflammation or infection may have other etiologies of symptoms such as small intestinal bacterial overgrowth, bile acid diarrhea, and irritable bowel disease.

H. Patients with confirmed active inflammation due to IBD may benefit from a course of corticosteroids to induce remission. At this time, it is possible to empirically increase the dose of biologic or decrease the dosing interval. However, it is preferable to perform drug monitoring to check trough drug level and presence of anti-drug antibodies to guide further management. This approach is called "*reactive therapeutic drug monitoring*." Trough levels should be checked just before scheduled administration of the drug.

I. If drug trough levels are low and anti-drug antibodies are high, then the biologic should be switched to another drug with the same MOA (e.g., infliximab to adalimumab). Concurrent immunosuppression will decrease the likelihood of immunogenicity for the second biologic. Other options include switching to another biologic with a different MOA (e.g., infliximab to vedolizumab), or in ulcerative colitis, switching to a small molecule.

J. If drug trough levels are low and anti-drug antibodies are negative or low, then the dose of the biologic should be increased, or the dosing interval decreased to try to achieve higher drug trough levels.

K. If drug trough levels are within the therapeutic range, then the biologic should be switched to another biologic with a different MOA. In ulcerative colitis, switching to a small molecule is another therapeutic option.

BIBLIOGRAPHY

1. Feuerstein JD, Ho EY, Shmidt E, et al. AGA clinical practice guidelines on the medical management of moderate to severe luminal and perianal fistulizing Crohn's disease. *Gastroenterology*. 2021;160(7):2496-2508. https://doi.org/10.1053/j.gastro.2021.04.022.
2. Singh S, Ananthakrishnan AN, Nguyen NH, et al. AGA clinical practice guideline on the role of biomarkers for the management of ulcerative colitis. *Gastroenterology*. 2023;164(3):344-372. https://doi.org/10.1053/j.gastro.2022.12.007.
3. Feuerstein JD, Nguyen GC, Kupfer SS, Falck-Ytter Y, Singh S, American Gastroenterological Association Institute Clinical Guidelines Committee. American Gastroenterological Association Institute guideline on therapeutic drug monitoring in inflammatory bowel disease. *Gastroenterology*. 2017;153(3):827-834. https://doi.org/10.1053/j.gastro.2017.07.032.

ALGORITHM 71.1 Flowchart for the approach to starting and switching biologic therapy for inflammatory bowel disease *(IBD)*. *CMV*, Cytomegalovirus; *CT*, computed tomography; *MOA*, mechanism of action; *MRE*, magnetic resonance enterography; *PPD*, purified protein derivative; *TB*, tuberculosis; *UC*, ulcerative colitis.

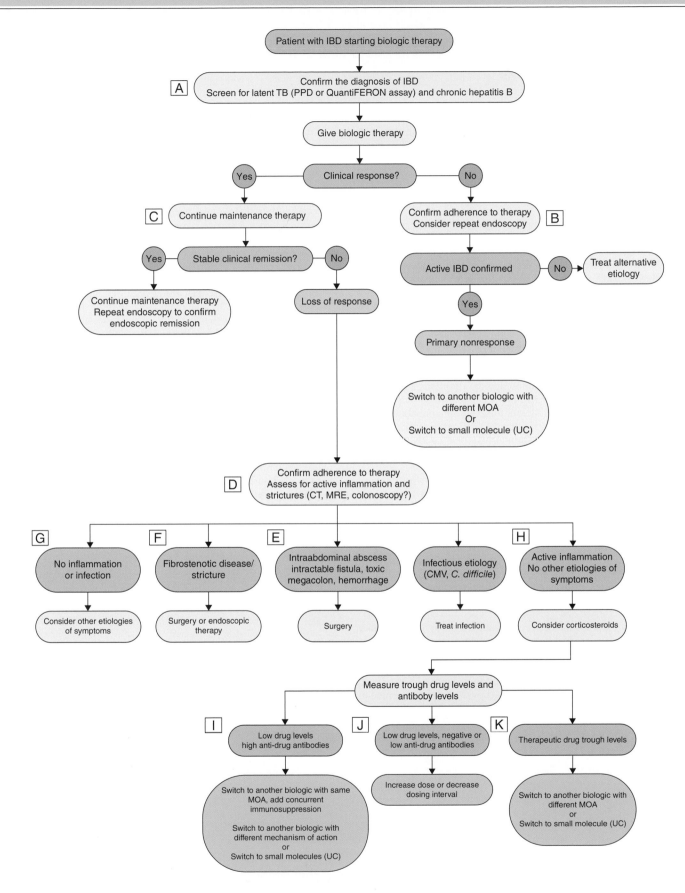

72 Surveillance of Colorectal Neoplasia in Inflammatory Bowel Disease

Nikrad Shahnavaz

Patients with inflammatory bowel disease (IBD) involving the colon have an increased risk of colorectal cancer (CRC), with the exception of those with isolated proctitis. The most important risk factor is duration of the disease, followed by presence of coexisting primary sclerosing cholangitis (PSC), extent of the colon involvement, and severity of inflammation. Other risk factors include family history of CRC, male gender, age at diagnosis of IBD, and possibly backwash ileitis.

A. The first screening colonoscopy for dysplasia should be performed immediately after diagnosis of PSC or 8–10 years after diagnosis of IBD in all patients with colonic involvement (except isolated proctitis). Targeted biopsies from suspicious mucosal findings, endoscopic resection of clearly demarcated lesions (without stigmata of invasive cancer or submucosal fibrosis), and extensive nontargeted biopsies (four quadrants biopsies every 10 cm) from flat colorectal mucosa are recommended when white light endoscopy is used. If dye spray or virtual (narrow band imaging) high-definition chromoendoscopy is used, performing extensive nontargeted biopsies of the normal mucosa is not necessary.

B. After a negative screening colonoscopy for dysplasia, surveillance colonoscopy should be performed every 1–5 years based on risk factors for CRC. Presence of moderate to severe inflammation of any extent, PSC, and strong family history of CRC will warrant surveillance colonoscopy in 1 year. Minimal historical colitis extent and previous consecutive examinations without dysplasia will indicate 5-year intervals.

C. Clearly delineated lesions without features of invasive cancer or submucosal fibrosis (mucosal depression, irregular surface architecture, radiating folds, or failure to lift with submucosal saline injection) should be resected endoscopically based on current guidelines. Small polypoid lesions could be safely removed with standard polypectomy techniques. Larger (>2 cm) complex (especially nonpolypoid) lesions are referred to endoscopists experienced in endoscopic mucosal resection (EMR) and endoscopic submucosal dissection (ESD).

D. After endoscopic resection of pedunculated polyps or lesions smaller than 1 cm with low-grade dysplasia, surveillance colonoscopy should be done in 2 years. Polyps with low-grade dysplasia, which are larger than 1 cm warrant surveillance in 1 year. If the lesion demonstrates any evidence of high-grade dysplasia or if there is any concern about complete resection, subsequent colonoscopy should be performed in 3–6 months.

E. If the surveillance colonoscopy demonstrates any evidence of incomplete resection or local recurrence of the dysplastic lesions, the options of repeat colonoscopy with second attempt at resection, surgery, or intensive surveillance need to be discussed with the patient and the surgery team.

F. Lesions deemed to be unresectable should be biopsied and then tattooed with India Ink stain placed at least 3 cm distal to the lesion and referred for surgery (partial or total colectomy).

G. If nontargeted biopsies from normal mucosa during surveillance colonoscopy reveal dysplasia, the first step is to confirm the findings by a second expert pathologist. Colonoscopy should be repeated by an experienced endoscopist using high-definition dye spray chromoendoscopy with the goal of uncovering subtle lesions for targeted resection as well as extensive nontargeted biopsies in the area of prior dysplasia, if no lesion is seen. Active colitis should be controlled before the second colonoscopy to avoid misdiagnosis of reactive atypia as dysplasia.

H. Persistent high-grade dysplasia or multifocal low-grade dysplasia are is highly predictive of concurrent or subsequent CRC, and colectomy is typically recommended for these patients.

I. For patients with unifocal low-grade dysplasia or no dysplasia found on the subsequent high-quality chromoendoscopy, current guidelines recommend intensive surveillance with chromoendoscopy with 6- to 12-month intervals until two consecutive negative high-quality examinations are documented. However, the long-term outcome of this approach is uncertain and risk-benefit discussion with patients regarding surgery versus surveillance is strongly recommended.

BIBLIOGRAPHY

1. Ananthakrishnan AN, Regueiro MD Management of Inflammatory bowel diseases. Sleisenger and Fordtran's Gastrointestinal and Liver Disease. 11th ed. Elsevier; 2020.
2. Rubin DT, Ananthakrishnan AN, Siegel CA, et al. ACG clinical guideline: ulcerative colitis in adults. *Am J Gastroenterol.* 2019;114(3):384-413.
3. Murthy SK, Feuerstein JD, Nguyen GC, et al. AGA clinical practice update on endoscopic surveillance and management of colorectal dysplasia in inflammatory bowel diseases: expert review. *Gastroenterology.* 2021;161(3):1043-1051. e4.

ALGORITHM 72.1 Surveillance of colorectal neoplasia in inflammatory bowel disease (*IBD*). *EMR*, Endoscopic mucosal resection; *ESD*, endoscopic submucosal dissection.

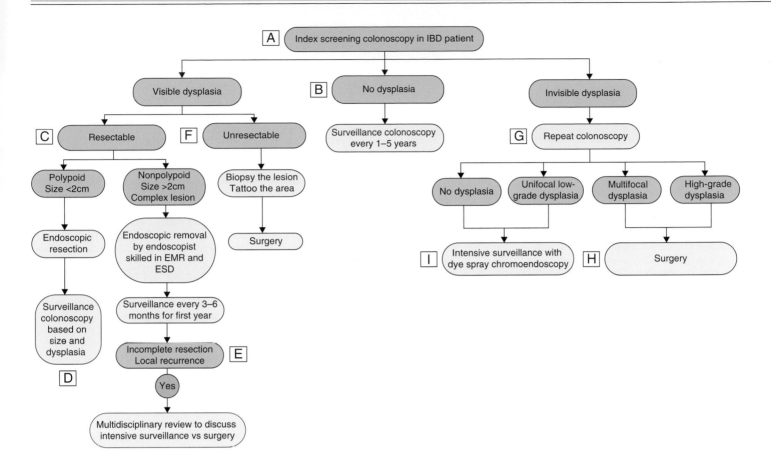

73 Colonic Ischemia

Emad Qayed

Colonic ischemia (CI) is the most common type of intestinal ischemic injury, and predominantly affects older adults. CI usually develops due to alteration in the systemic circulation leading to mesenteric hypoperfusion (i.e., nonocclusive ischemia), or due to acute arterial occlusion from thrombosis or embolus. Depending on the severity of CI, the colon may develop transient colitis, chronic colitis, stricture, gangrene, and fulminant pancolitis.

A. The diagnosis of CI is suspected from the clinical evaluation, based on symptoms, signs, and risk factors. Patients present with sudden onset abdominal pain associated with fecal urgency and hematochezia. Medical comorbidities associated with CI include atherosclerosis, atrial fibrillation, heart failure, diabetes, hypertension, and peripheral vascular disease. Vasculitis, coagulation disorders, and illicit drugs (e.g., cocaine) are usually the cause of CI in young patients. A complete list of possible etiologies for CI is presented in Boxes 73.1 and 73.2. In patients with severe ischemic colitis or gangrene, physical examination may reveal signs of peritonitis such as abdominal rigidity, guarding, and rebound tenderness.

B. The initial workup of a patient with suspected CI should begin with laboratory studies including complete blood cell count, renal and hepatic panels, lactate dehydrogenase (LDH), and lactate levels. In patients with diarrhea, stool studies should be obtained to rule out infectious diarrhea such as *Clostridioides difficile* infection. All patients should receive supportive care, with a search for underlying etiology or medications. Patients with signs of sepsis should receive broad-spectrum antibiotics.

C. The imaging test of choice in patients with suspected CI is computed tomography (CT) scan of the abdomen and pelvis with intravenous (IV) contrast. Further management depends on the findings of initial assessment and CT scan.

D. Patients with peritoneal signs on physical examination, pneumatosis, portal venous gas, or pancolonic involvement are considered to have severe CI. These patients should be transferred to the intensive care unit, given broad-spectrum antibiotics, and evaluated emergently by the surgical service. Acute indications for surgery in CI include peritoneal signs, massive bleeding, fulminant colitis, portal venous gas, pneumatosis intestinalis, or gangrenous bowel on colonoscopy, or any patients with deteriorating clinical course. The type of surgery depends on the location and extent of ischemia, and may include total or subtotal colectomy, right hemicolectomy, or segmental colectomy.

E. For isolated right-sided CI (IRCI), CT angiography (CTA), magnetic resonance angiography (MRA), or conventional direct angiography should be performed to evaluate for focal occlusion in the superior mesenteric artery. If there is vascular occlusion, treatment may include anticoagulation, intraarterial perfusion with vasodilators or thrombolytic agents, endovascular intervention, or surgical revascularization.

F. Patients with CT findings consistent with CI but without severe findings are further categorized based on the presence of risk factors for severe disease. These include male sex, hypotension (systolic blood pressure [SBP] < 90 mm Hg), tachycardia [heart rate (HR) > 100 beats per minute], abdominal pain without rectal bleeding, white blood cell (WBC) >15 × 10^9/L, hemoglobin (Hgb) <12 g/dL, blood urea nitrogen (BUN) >20 mg/dL, serum sodium <136 mmol/L, LDH >350 U/L. If there are more than three of these risk factors, then the patient is considered to have severe CI.

G. Colonoscopy and biopsy should be considered in all patients without features of severe disease, and in some patients with severe disease in which symptoms improve but do not resolve, or if the diagnosis is still unclear. The goal of colonoscopy is to rule out alternative diagnoses and establish the severity of ischemia. The procedure should be performed with gentle insertion and insufflation. The colonoscope does not need to reach the cecum if there are severe ischemic changes in the left colon.

H. If there are no ulcerations, antibiotics can be discontinued, while patients with CI and ulcerations should receive antibiotics. If colonoscopy reveals signs of IRCI, workup with CTA, MRA, or conventional angiography should be considered. If gangrenous bowel is seen during colonoscopy, this requires immediate surgery.

I. Patients with CI require follow-up to ensure healing without complications. Long-term complications of CI include recurrent abdominal pain, diarrhea, sepsis due to bacteremia, and colonic strictures.

BIBLIOGRAPHY

1. Sleisenger and Fordtran's Gastrointestinal and Liver Disease, 11th Edition, Elsevier, 2021. Chapter 73, Colonic Ischemia.
2. Brandt LJ, Feuerstadt P, Longstreth GF, et al. American College of Gastroenterology. ACG clinical guideline: epidemiology, risk factors, patterns of presentation, diagnosis, and management of colon ischemia (CI). *Am J Gastroenterol.* 2015;110(1):18-44. quiz 45.

ALGORITHM 73.1 Flowchart for the workup of suspected colonic ischemia *(CI)*. *Risk factors for severe disease: male sex, hypotension (SBP <90 mm Hg), tachycardia (HR >100 beats per minute), abdominal pain without rectal bleeding, WBC >15 × 10^9/L, Hgb <12 g/dL, BUN >20 mg/dL, serum sodium <136 mmol/L, LDH >350 U/L. *BUN*: blood urea nitrogen; *CBC*: complete blood count; *CTA*: computed tomography angiography; *Hgb*: hemoglobin; *HR*: heart rate; *IRCI*: isolated right-sided colonic ischemia; *IV*, intravenous; *LDH*: lactate dehydrogenase; *MRA*: magnetic resonance angiography; *SBP*: systolic blood pressure; *WBC*: white blood cell.

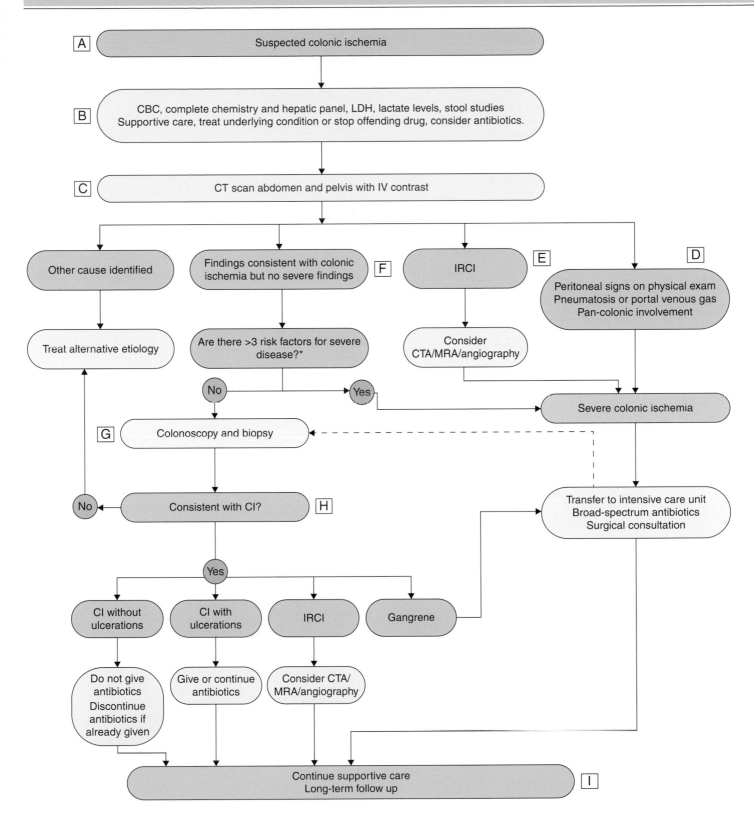

A Suspected colonic ischemia

B CBC, complete chemistry and hepatic panel, LDH, lactate levels, stool studies
Supportive care, treat underlying condition or stop offending drug, consider antibiotics.

C CT scan abdomen and pelvis with IV contrast

Other cause identified

Findings consistent with colonic ischemia but no severe findings   F

IRCI   E

D Peritoneal signs on physical exam
Pneumatosis or portal venous gas
Pan-colonic involvement

Treat alternative etiology

Are there >3 risk factors for severe disease?*

Consider CTA/MRA/angiography

No   Yes

Severe colonic ischemia

G Colonoscopy and biopsy

No   Consistent with CI?   H

Transfer to intensive care unit
Broad-spectrum antibiotics
Surgical consultation

Yes

CI without ulcerations

CI with ulcerations

IRCI

Gangrene

Do not give antibiotics
Discontinue antibiotics if already given

Give or continue antibiotics

Consider CTA/MRA/angiography

Continue supportive care
Long-term follow up   I

BOX 73.1 CAUSES OF COLONIC ISCHEMIA

Acute pancreatitis

Allergy

Amyloidosis

Heart failure or cardiac arrhythmias

Hematologic disorders and coagulopathies
  Activated protein C resistance
  Antithrombin deficiency
  Paroxysmal nocturnal hemoglobinuria
  Polycythemia vera
  Protein C and S deficiencies
  Prothrombin G20210A mutation
  Sickle cell disease

Infection
  Bacteria (*Escherichia coli* O157:H7)
  Parasites (*Angiostrongylus costaricensis*)
  Viruses (hepatitis B and C, HCV, CMV)

Inferior mesenteric artery thrombosis

Long-distance running and flying

Medications and toxins (see Box 73.2 for details)
  Antibiotics
  Appetite suppressants
  Chemotherapy
  Constipation-inducing medications
  Decongestants
  Diuretics
  Ergot alkaloids
  Hormonal therapies
  Illicit drugs
  Immunomodulators
  Interferon
  Laxatives

NSAIDs
Serotonin agents
Statins
Vasopressor agents

Pheochromocytoma

Ruptured ectopic pregnancy

Shock

Strangulated hernia

Surgery/procedures
  Aortic aneurysmectomy
  Aortoiliac reconstruction
  Barium enema
  Colectomy with inferior mesenteric artery ligation
  Colon bypass
  Colonoscopy
  Exchange transfusions
  Gynecologic operations
  Lumbar aortography

Thromboembolism
  Cholesterol (atheroembolism)
  Myxoma (left atrial)

Trauma (blunt or penetrating)

Vasculitis and vasculopathy
  Buerger disease
  Fibromuscular dysplasia
  Kawasaki disease
  Polyarteritis nodosa
  Rheumatoid vasculitis
  SLE
  Takayasu arteritis

Volvulus

CMV, Cytomegalovirus; *HCV*, hepatitis C virus; *NSAID*, nonsteroidal antiinflammatory drugs; *SLE*, systemic lupus erythematosus.

BOX 73.2 MEDICATIONS AND TOXINS ASSOCIATED WITH COLONIC ISCHAEMIA

Antibiotics
  Fluoroquinolones
  Penicillin and penicillin derivatives

Appetite suppressants
  Hydroxycut
  Phentermine

Chemotherapy
  Platinum-based therapy
  Taxanes
  Vinorelbine

Constipation-inducing medications
  Antipsychotics (e.g., alosetron, quetiapine,
    clozapine)
  Opioid agonists (e.g., loperamide, oxycodone,
    hydrocodone, morphine, codeine)
  Muscarinic agonists (e.g., diphenhydramine,
    dicyclomine)

Decongestants
  Phenylephrine
  Pseudoephedrine

Diuretics
  Furosemide

Ergot alkaloids
  Dihydroergotamine mesylate

Hormonal therapies
  OCP (e.g., ethinyl estradiol and desogestrel,
    drospirenone and ethinyl estradiol,
    levonorgestrel-ethinyl-estradiol)
  Vaginal rings (e.g., etonogestrel, ethinylestradiol)

Illicit drugs
  Amphetamines
  Cocaine

Immunomodulators
  Glucocorticoids
  Lenalinomide
  TNF-α inhibitors

Interferon

Laxatives
  Bisacodyl
  Glycerin enema
  Magnesium citrate
  Polyethylene glycol
  Sevelamer
  Sodium phosphate
  Sodium polystyrene sulfonate

NSAIDs/low-dose ASA

Serotonin agents
  Alosetron
  Clozapine
  Quetiapine
  Sumatriptan

Statins
  Rosuvastatin
  Simvastatin

Vasopressor agents
  Glypressin
  Vasopressin

Others
  Danazol
  Flutamide
  Gold salts
  Pit viper toxin

ASA, Acetylsalicylic acid; *NSAIDs*, nonsteroidal antiinflammatory drugs; *OCP*, oral contraceptive; *TNF*, tumor necrosis factor.

74 | Immune Checkpoint Inhibitors Colitis

Elnaz Jafarimehr

Immune checkpoint inhibitors (ICIs) revolutionized treatment and survival of patients with different cancers including small-cell lung cancer, renal cell carcinoma, and melanoma. By targeting immune checkpoints involving in downregulation of cytotoxic T cells, ICIs promote cytotoxic T-cell survival, and its antitumor action.

They also activate global T-cell response and induce immune-related adverse events including immune-mediated colitis. The incidence of colitis for patients using antiprogrammed cell death protein 1 (PD-1) is 0.7%–1.6% while the incidence for patients using anticytotoxic T lymphocyte–associated protein 4 (CTLA-4) is 5.7%–9.1%, and 13.6% with combination therapy. Examples of ICI include Ipilimumab, tremelimumab, nivolumab, cemiplimab, pembrolizumab, atezolizumab, avelumab, and durvalumab.

A. The American Society of Clinical Oncology defines both diarrhea and colitis based on symptomatic presentation.

Grade 1: Increase of <4 stools/day over baseline and patients are asymptomatic

Grade 2: Increase of 4–6 stools/day and patients could have abdominal pain, mucous, and blood in the stools

Grade 3: Increase of ≥7 stools/day and patient may feel severe pain, fever, peritoneal signs, and ileus

Grade 4: Patients may have life-threatening consequences including intestinal perforation, ischemia, necrosis, and toxic megacolon

In any patients with chronic diarrhea and suspected ICI colitis, laboratory tests should be considered including complete blood count, complete metabolic panel, celiac serology, C-reactive protein, cytomegalovirus, thyroid stimulating hormone, lipase, and amylase. In addition, stool tests should be sent for stool culture, ova and parasite, and *Clostridioides difficile* nucleic acid amplification test. Other tests to be considered are fecal lactoferrin, calprotectin, fecal pancreatic elastase, and multiplex polymerase chain reaction panels to check for infectious etiologies. Patients should be screened for human immunodeficiency syndrome (HIV), tuberculosis (Quantiferon-TB gold), and viral hepatitis A, B, and C. Infection with the fungi Histoplasma *capsulatum* can lead to disseminated disease with inflammatory diarrhea similar to inflammatory bowel disease; therefore, checking urine histoplasma antigen can be considered. Gastrointestinal (GI) consultation for ileocolonoscopy or flexible sigmoidoscopy with biopsy is needed if symptoms are consistent with grade ≥2, or if persistent grade 1 despite conservative management, or with positive fecal inflammatory markers. Also, consider upper endoscopy with ≥grade 3 toxicity, persistent grade 2 symptoms, or atypical symptoms. Abdominal/pelvis computed tomography (CT) scan with contrast is indicated if there is any concern for toxic megacolon or perforation.

B. Supportive care is recommended for grade 1 diarrhea. Patients could consider bland diet and symptoms of diarrhea should be managed with antimotility agents (e.g., loperamide) and hydration. Treatment with ICIs could be continued.

C. Hospitalization is advised for patients with grade 2 symptoms if the patient has dehydration, fever, and systemic symptoms. Such patients would benefit from starting systemic corticosteroids such as prednisone at an initial dose of 1 mg/kg/day. Steroid tapering over 4–6 weeks is advised if symptoms improve to grade 1. If symptoms fail to improve after 48–72 hours, increasing the corticosteroid dose to prednisone 2 mg/kg/day or switching to intravenous methylprednisolone sodium succinate is recommended. Alternatively, clinicians may switch to biologics with infliximab or vedolizumab if no improvement in symptoms after 2–3 days is seen. Hold treatment with ICIs but consider permanent discontinuation of anti-CTLA 4 agents.

D. Hospitalization is advised for patients with grade 3 diarrhea with dehydration or systemic symptoms. Corticosteroids are administered at an initial dose of 1–2 mg/kg/day of prednisone or equivalents. If symptoms improve to grade 1 or less, the patient should be switched to an oral prednisone taper over at least 4–6 weeks. Increase the dose of corticosteroids or switch to biologics if there is no improvement in the symptoms after 2 to 3 days similar to patients with grade 2. Biologics should be considered if there is incomplete response within a week, or if the patient has recurrent symptoms during tapering period or after completion of treatment. Biologics are also recommended if colonoscopy demonstrates colonic ulcerations. ICIs should be withheld, but consider permanent discontinuation of anti-CTLA-4 agents.

E. In patients with grade 4 symptoms and colitis, treatment of ICIs should be permanently discontinued. Hospitalization is required for all patients with grade 4 colitis. Start treatment with intravenous methylprednisolone at 1–2 mg/kg/day until symptoms improve to grade 1 or less. If symptoms persist after 2–3 days of corticosteroid treatment or if ulcers are noted during colonoscopy, prompt administration of biologics should be considered. If patients do not improve on biologic therapy, consider high- dose infliximab, fecal microbiota transplantation (as part of a clinical trial), or colectomy.

BIBLIOGRAPHY

1. Abu-Sbeih H, Faleck DM, Ricciuti B, et al. Immune checkpoint inhibitor therapy in patients with preexisting inflammatory bowel disease. *J Clin Oncol.* 2020;38(6):576-583.
2. Powell N, Ibraheim H, Raine T, et al. British Society of Gastroenterology endorsed guidance for the management of immune checkpoint inhibitor-induced enterocolitis. *Lancet Gastroenterol Hepatol.* 2020;5(7):679-697.
3. Bellaguarda E, Hanauer S. Checkpoint inhibitor-induced colitis. *Am J Gastroenterol.* 2020;115(2):202-210.
4. Hashash J, Francis F, Farraye F. Diagnosis and management of immune checkpoint inhibitor colitis. *Gastroenterol Hepatol (N Y).* 2021;17(8):358-366.
5. Hamdeh S, Micic D, Hanauer S. Drug-induced colitis. *Clin Gastroenterol Hepatol.* 2021;19(9):1759-1779. https://doi.org/10.1016/j.cgh.2020.04.069.

ALGORITHM 74.1 Flowchart for the management of immune checkpoint inhibitors colitis. *ICI,* Immune checkpoint inhibitors; *IV,* intravenous.

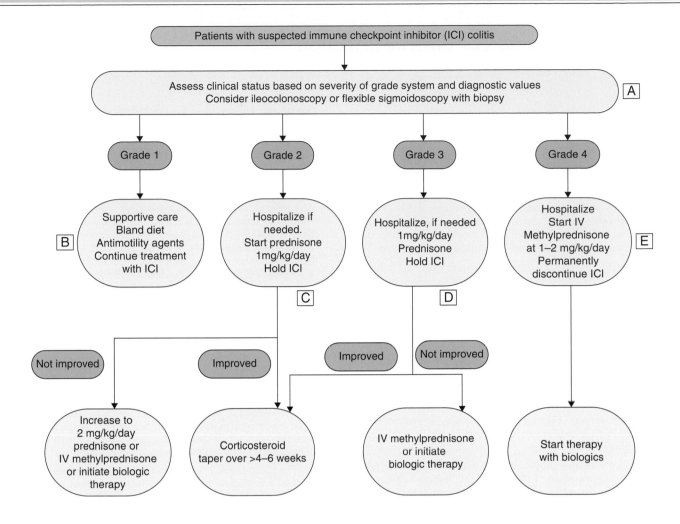

75 *Clostridioides difficile* Infection

Thuy-Van Pham Hang

Clostridioides difficile infection (CDI) occurs when this Gram-positive bacterium produces toxin A or B, which leads to colonic inflammation and diarrhea. Risk factors for CDI include contact with the healthcare environment, age ≥65 years, antibiotic use, White race, cardiac disease, chronic kidney disease, and inflammatory bowel disease. Colonization with *C. difficile* is a common phenomenon in which the organism is detected but the patient is *without* symptoms; this can occur up to 21% of hospitalized adults and is *not* considered synonymous with CDI. Predictors of poor outcomes include severe or fulminant CDI, low albumin, fecal calprotectin >2000 mcg/g, peripheral eosinophilia or undetectable eosinophils, fever >38.5°C, and pseudomembranes on colonoscopy.

A. Testing for CDI occurs in a two-step process involving a highly sensitive then highly specific testing modality to help differentiate colonization from CDI. Glutamate dehydrogenase (GDH) antigen testing identifies the presence of this enzyme, which is made by both toxigenic and nontoxigenic *Clostridioides* strains. Nucleic acid amplification testing (NAAT) uses polymerase chain reaction (PCR) or loop-mediated isothermal amplification to identify the presence of a toxigenic strain but cannot determine if it is producing toxins or not. GDH and NAAT are both very sensitive tests with high negative predictive values. If there is high suspicion for CDI in a patient with ileus and no diarrhea, a rectal swab for PCR can be used.

B. Enzyme immunoassay (EIA) tests are highly specific and can detect toxins A and B. The sensitivity of EIA testing can be affected by specimen handling.

C. Three different scenarios should be considered with a positive GDH or NAAT then negative toxin EIA testing: (1) *C. difficile* colonization, (2) false negative toxin EIA, or (3) toxin levels are below the threshold of detection. If there is high clinical suspicion for CDI, empiric treatment should still be pursued.

D. Nonsevere and severe CDI can be treated with 10 days of either oral vancomycin 125 mg four times daily or oral fidaxomicin 200 mg twice daily. In cases of nonsevere CDI in low-risk patients (young outpatients with minimal comorbidities), oral metronidazole 500 mg three times daily can be utilized. Metronidazole should *not* be used in the case of severe CDI given inferiority compared to vancomycin in multiple randomized control trials and cohort studies. In patients with underlying inflammatory bowel disease, vancomycin 125 mg four times daily for a minimum of 14 days is preferred. Vancomycin is preferred in pregnant, peripartum, and breastfeeding patients. Antimotility agents should not be used in untreated CDI given risk of toxic megacolon but can be added as needed after antibiotics are initiated for cases of nonsevere and severe CDI. Bile acid–binding agents like cholestyramine should not be used, as these can bind antibiotics. Psyllium and fiber can be safely added on during the recovery phase. If there is an appropriate indication for antisecretory treatment (i.e., proton pump inhibitors), they should be continued.

E. For patients with fulminant CDI, in addition to adequate volume resuscitation, treatment should be initiated with higher dose oral vancomycin 500 mg every 6 hours for the first 48–72 hours, followed by oral vancomycin 125 mg four times daily for 10 days if there is clinical improvement. The addition of parenteral metronidazole (500 mg in 100 mL saline) every 8 hours should be considered. Vancomycin enemas 500 mg every 6 hours should be added for patients with ileus. There should be a low threshold for cross-sectional imaging to determine the severity of CDI and detect the presence of megacolon or perforation. Antimotility agents should be avoided in cases of fulminant CDI.

F. If surgical intervention is pursued, either a total colectomy with end ileostomy and a stapled rectal stump or a diverting loop ileostomy with colonic lavage and intraluminal vancomycin is recommended. Fecal microbiota transplantation (FMT) should be considered in cases of medically refractory severe and fulminant CDI, especially if the patient is a poor surgical candidate. While a majority of patients will respond to one FMT, many require multiple FMTs to be cured from CDI. FMT should be repeated every 3–5 days until pseudomembranes are no longer seen, during which the final FMT would be performed. Concurrent oral antibiotics with either vancomycin or fidaxomicin should be continued until no pseudomembranes are detected. If the patient is discharged before resolution of pseudomembranes, oral antibiotics should be continued for at least another 5 days, followed by a final outpatient FMT.

G. Recurrent CDI (rCDI) occurs when there is recurrent diarrhea with positive NAAT or EIA within 8 weeks after the treatment of an initial episode of CDI. This can occur in approximately 20% of patients. Treatment options depend on the antibiotic course the patient received during their index infection. A tapering/pulse dose vancomycin course (oral vancomycin 125 mg four times daily for 10–14 days then twice daily for 7 days then daily for 7 days, then every 2–3 days for 2–8 weeks) can be used no matter which antibiotic was used initially. If fidaxomicin was *not* used during the initial course, it can be used to treat rCDI at a dose of 200 mg twice daily for 10 days. The use of metronidazole is not recommended in rCDI.

H. FMT is recommended for second rCDI or subsequent recurrences to prevent further recurrences. Two fecal microbiota products are approved by the Food and Drug Administration (FDA) to be given to patients with one or more recurrences of CDI. However, most physicians will try FMT after the second recurrence. They are administered after completion of antibiotic treatment for the rCDI episode. These products are packaged in suspension form for rectal administration, and in capsule forms for oral administration. If the patient is not an FMT candidate, long-term suppressive oral vancomycin can be used. FMT is not recommended in pregnancy given procedural risks and lack of data. Immunocompromised patients should undergo screening for cytomegalovirus and Epstein–Barr virus before FMT given the transmission risk.

I. Patients should be evaluated within a week of the procedure to assess for recurrence or adverse events. They should then be reevaluated 4–8 weeks post-FMT to identify late FMT failure. Once FMT failure is identified, anti-CDI antibiotics should be restarted. Repeat FMT is indicated for those who experience rCDI within 8 weeks of their initial FMT. If FMT was received via enema or capsules, colonoscopic delivery should be performed during the repeat FMT. If the patient does not want to or cannot undergo repeat FMT, a prolonged or indefinite oral vancomycin course (tapered down to 125 mg daily) can be used. Probiotics are *not* recommended for prevention of recurrence.

BIBLIOGRAPHY

1. Kelly CR, Fischer M, Allegretti JR, et al. ACG clinical guidelines: prevention, diagnosis, and treatment of *Clostridioides difficile* infections. *Am J Gastroenterol.* 2021;116(6):1124-1147. Erratum in: *Am J Gastroenterol.* 2022;117(2):358.
2. Johnson S, Lavergne V, Skinner AM, et al. Clinical practice guideline by the Infectious Diseases Society of America (IDSA) and Society for Healthcare Epidemiology of America (SHEA): 2021 focused update guidelines on management of *Clostridioides difficile* infection in adults. *Clinical Infectious Diseases.* 2021;73(5):755-757.

ALGORITHM 75.1 Flowchart for the diagnosis and management of *Clostridioides difficile* infection. *BMP,* Basic metabolic panel; *CBC,* complete blood count; *CDI, Clostridioides difficile* infection; *Cr,* creatinine; *EIA,* enzyme immunoassay; *FMT,* fecal microbiota transplantation; *GDH,* glutamate dehydrogenase; *IV,* intravenous; *NAAT,* nucleic acid amplification testing; *PO,* per oral; *PR,* per rectum; *WBC,* white blood cell.

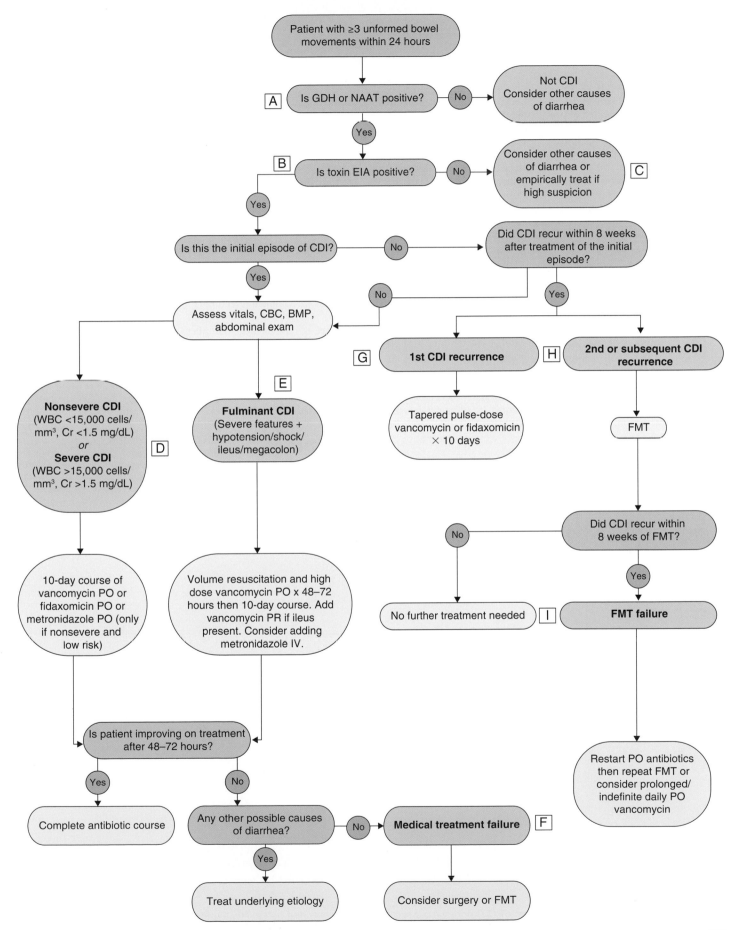

Colon Polyp Surveillance

Nikrad Shahnavaz

When colonoscopy is performed for colorectal cancer (CRC) screening, the colonoscopist is expected to provide the patient and referring physician with follow-up recommendations on the need for surveillance colonoscopy and its timing in the future. The risk of metachronous advanced polyps and neoplasia is associated with findings on index colonoscopy. The US Multi-Society Task Force released its latest recommendations for postcolonoscopy follow-up and polyp surveillance in 2020.

A. CRC screening is recommended to be started at the age of 45 years in individuals with average risk and to be continued at least through age 75 years, or as long as the life expectancy is 10 years or longer. Colonoscopy is the preferred test for CRC screening.

B. Patients are categorized as having "average risk for CRC" when they do *not* have any of the following conditions: personal history of CRC, inflammatory bowel disease, family history of CRC, hereditary syndrome associated with increased CRC risk, or serrated polyposis syndrome. Individuals with "high risk" for CRC may need to initiate CRC screening at younger age and repeat it in shorter intervals based on guidelines for each different condition.

C. High-quality colonoscopy is defined as an examination complete to cecum with adequate bowel preparation (to reliably detect lesions >5 mm) performed by colonoscopist with adequate adenoma detection rate (>30% in men; >20% in women), and attention to complete polyp excision.

D. A colonoscopy is considered "normal" (with no polyps) when no adenoma, sessile serrated polyp (SSP), traditional serrated adenoma (TSA), hyperplastic polyp (HP) larger than 10 mm, or CRC is found.

E. Adenomas and SSPs are now classified as neoplastic polyps, although HPs (early stage of serrated lesions) are considered nonneoplastic. SSPs are a heterogeneous group of lesions that are distinguished from conventional adenomas primarily by a saw-tooth or stellate appearance of their colonic crypts. Nonneoplastic polyps such as hamartomatous, inflammatory, or mucosal prolapse polyps found during the screening colonoscopy will not shorten the recommended interval for surveillance colonoscopy.

F. Advanced adenoma is an adenoma with one or more of the following findings: (1) >10 mm in size, (2) adenoma with tubulovillous/villous histology, and (3) adenoma with high-grade dysplasia.

G. Piecemeal resection of adenomas ≥20 mm in size should be followed by a repeat endoscopy to examine the polypectomy site in 6 months to ensure complete resection.

H. There is no evidence to confirm increased risk for metachronous advanced neoplasia or large serrated polyps among patients with isolated HPs <10 mm found either proximal or distal to the sigmoid colon. However, if there is concern regarding the ability of the local pathologist to distinguish between SSP and HPs, the colonoscopist may choose to follow the recommendations for SSPs for patients identified with isolated proximal HPs <10 mm.

BIBLIOGRAPHY

1. Gupta S, Lieberman D, Anderson JC, et al. Recommendations for follow-up after colonoscopy and polypectomy: a consensus update by the US Multi-Society Task Force on Colorectal Cancer. *Gastroenterology.* 2020;158(4): 1131-1153.

ALGORITHM 76.1 Colon polyp surveillance. *CRC,* Colorectal cancer; *SSP,* sessile serrated polyp; *HP,* hyperplastic polyp.

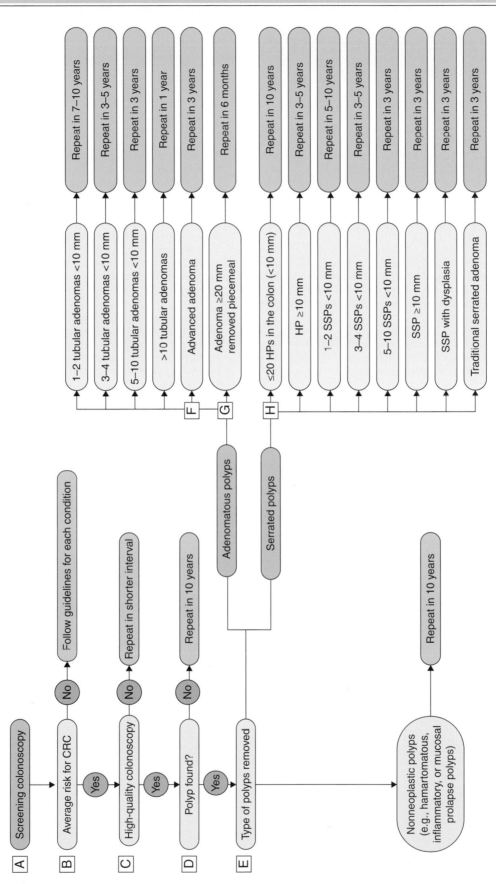

77 Malignant Colorectal Polyps

Emad Qayed

The term *malignant polyp* refers to an adenomatous polyp with a focus of carcinoma invading beyond the muscularis mucosa and into the submucosa. This corresponds to a T1 colorectal cancer tumor depth of invasion, based on the TNM staging by the American Joint Committee on Cancer (AJCC). A malignant polyp is also referred to as "*submucosally invasive lesion.*" It is important to differentiate these polyps from advanced polyps that contain intraepithelial or intramucosal carcinoma without submucosal invasion. This algorithm addresses isk of lymph node metastasis the management strategies of advanced and malignant polyps.

A. The presence of a malignancy within a polyp can be suspected by the endoscopist before resection of the polyp. When appropriate, these polyps should be resected en bloc with endoscopic mucosal resection or endoscopic submucosal dissection, and the site of polypectomy should be tattooed.

B. Once the polyp is removed endoscopically, careful histologic examination should be performed to identify presence of malignancy, depth of invasion, and other histologic features.

C. Polyps with high-grade dysplasia are considered advanced polyps. If resection is complete, then follow-up is with colonoscopy at 3 years.

D. Polyps with carcinoma in situ, defined as intraepithelial or intramucosal carcinoma, but without submucosal invasion, are also considered advanced polyps and not "malignant polyps." The risk of lymph node metastasis in these polyps is ~0%. Therefore they are managed similar to a polyp with high-grade dysplasia. Colonoscopy in 3 years is appropriate.

E. If the polyp contains malignant cells with submucosal invasion, but not extending into the muscularis propria, this is considered a malignant polyp.

F. The first step is to confirm that the polyp was completely resected endoscopically. If the polyp was not completely resected, then referral to surgical resection is appropriate. If the polyp has not been tattooed, then the endoscopy should be repeated to tattoo the polypectomy site.

G. The next step is to examine histology for unfavorable histologic features that are associated with lymph node metastasis. In addition to the listed features, some studies found that the histologic finding of tumor budding is associated with increased risk of lymph node metastasis. Tumor budding is seen as single tumor cells or clusters of up to four cells at the invasive margin of the cancer. If any of these features is present, the patient should be referred to surgery for colectomy and removal of regional lymph nodes. If a sessile malignant polyp was removed but the specimen is fragmented, the margins cannot be assessed, and polypectomy is considered inadequate.

H. If none of these high-risk features are present, then endoscopic polypectomy is considered adequate, and surveillance colonoscopy is performed in 1 year. The National Comprehensive Cancer Network guidelines mention that surgery can still be offered to patients with malignant sessile polyps even if they do not have unfavorable histologic features, because some studies found higher incidence of residual disease, recurrent disease, mortality, and hematogenous metastasis in patients with malignant sessile polyps compared to malignant pedunculated polyps. This is likely related to the higher rate of inadequate resection in malignant sessile polyps.

BIBLIOGRAPHY

1. Shaukat A, Kaltenbach T, Dominitz JA, et al. Endoscopic recognition and management strategies for malignant colorectal polyps: recommendations of the US Multi-Society Task Force on Colorectal Cancer. *Am J Gastroenterol.* 2020;115(11):1751-1767.
2. National Comprehensive Cancer Network. NCCN Clinical Practice Guidelines in Oncology (NCCN Guidelines®), Colon cancer (Version 1.2022); 2022 [accessed 07.08.22]. https://www.nccn.org/guidelines/nccn-guidelines.
3. Lugli A, Kirsch R, Ajioka Y, et al. Recommendations for reporting tumor budding in colorectal cancer based on the International Tumor Budding Consensus Conference (ITBCC) 2016. *Mod Pathol.* 2017;30(9):1299-1311. https://doi.org/10.1038/modpathol.2017.46.

ALGORITHM 77.1 Flowchart for the management of advanced and malignant colorectal polyps.

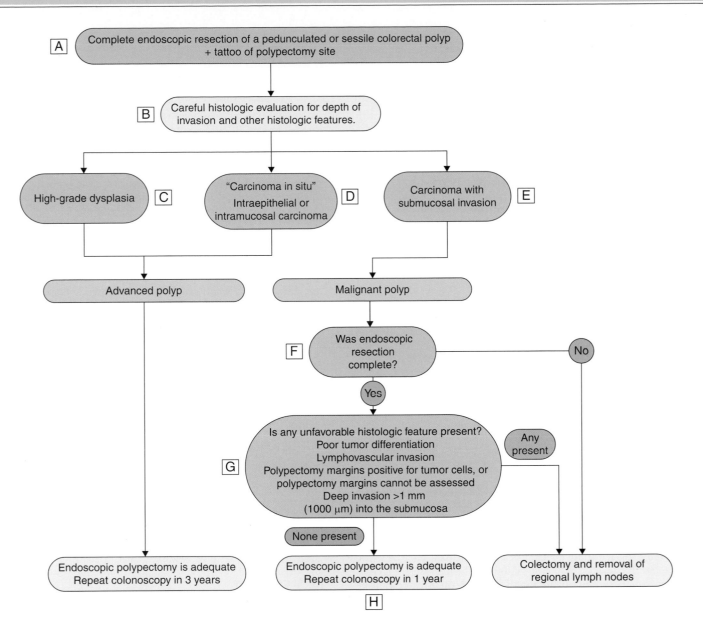

A — Complete endoscopic resection of a pedunculated or sessile colorectal polyp + tattoo of polypectomy site

B — Careful histologic evaluation for depth of invasion and other histologic features.

C — High-grade dysplasia

D — "Carcinoma in situ" Intraepithelial or intramucosal carcinoma

E — Carcinoma with submucosal invasion

Advanced polyp

Malignant polyp

F — Was endoscopic resection complete?

No

Yes

G — Is any unfavorable histologic feature present?
Poor tumor differentiation
Lymphovascular invasion
Polypectomy margins positive for tumor cells, or polypectomy margins cannot be assessed
Deep invasion >1 mm (1000 μm) into the submucosa

Any present

None present

Endoscopic polypectomy is adequate
Repeat colonoscopy in 3 years

H — Endoscopic polypectomy is adequate
Repeat colonoscopy in 1 year

Colectomy and removal of regional lymph nodes

78 Lynch Syndrome

Nikrad Shahnavaz

Lynch syndrome (LS) is an autosomal dominant disorder with colorectal and other organ malignancy as the major clinical consequence. LS is the most common hereditary colon cancer syndrome. The lifetime risk of colorectal cancer (CRC) in LS is dependent on the type of mismatch repair (MMR) gene, with higher risk for *MLH1* and *MSH2* gene mutation carriers compared to *MSH6* and *PMS2* mutations. Compared to sporadic CRC, patients with LS tend to have colon cancer diagnosed at younger age (mean age 45 years), and tumors are more likely to be located proximal to the splenic flexure. Also, multiple synchronous or metachronous colon cancers are more prevalent in patients with LS. On the other hand, tumors with microsatellite instability (MSI) have a more favorable prognosis compared to microsatellite-stable (MSS) tumors.

A. Universal testing for LS on the tumor biopsy specimen is currently recommended for all newly diagnosed CRCs, preferably before surgery. The alternative approach is selective strategy in which testing for LS is performed in patients diagnosed with colon cancer at age younger than 70 years, or older patients meeting any criteria of the revised Bethesda guidelines:
   1. CRC diagnosed at younger than 50 years.
   2. Presence of synchronous or metachronous CRC or other LS-associated tumors (endometrium, ovary, small bowel, stomach, hepatobiliary, brain, or urinary tract cancers).
   3. CRC with MSI-high pathologic-associated features (Crohn-like lymphocytic reaction, mucinous/signet cell differentiation, or medullary growth pattern) diagnosed in an individual younger than 60 years old.
   4. Patient with CRC and CRC or LS-associated tumor diagnosed in at least one first-degree relative younger than 50 years old.
   5. Patient with CRC and CRC or LS-associated tumor at any age in two first-degree or second-degree relatives.

B. The most specific study for LS is detecting the deficiency of MMR proteins. This can be achieved by immunohistochemistry (IHC), which entails staining of tumor tissue for protein expression of four MMR genes: *MLH1*, *MSH2*, *MSH6*, and *PMS2*. Abnormal expression of these gene products may indicate an underlying germline pathogenic variant. Alternatively, polymerase chain reaction (PCR) is used to measure the number of microsatellites in DNA from cancer cells to assess for MSI. MSI is the hallmark of LS-related malignancies. No further germline testing is necessary for MSS tumors.

C. Aberrant MLH1 gene promoter methylation is a somatic event that is limited to the CRC and is not inherited. It is responsible for causing loss of *MLH1* protein expression and results in MSI found in about 12% of sporadic CRCs. In addition, somatic BRAF V600 mutations have been detected predominantly in sporadic CRC. Consequently, the presence of a BRAF mutation or *MLH1* gene promoter hypermethylation in a patient with MSI-high CRC is evidence against the presence of LS.

D. Patients with abnormal IHC for *MSH2*, *MSH6*, *PMS2*, or *MLH1* (without BRAF mutation or *MLH1* gene promoter hypermethylation) should be referred to genetic counseling for germline testing guided by IHC testing results. Germline testing for MMR gene mutations is necessary to confidently diagnose LS. Before germline testing, patients should undergo genetic counseling to discuss the benefits and implications of identifying a germline mutation, both for the patient and the family.

E. After LS is diagnosed with germline testing, the patient should start surveillance for CRC (colonoscopy every 1–2 years), endometrial/ovarian cancer (annual pelvic examination with endometrial sampling and transvaginal ultrasound), gastric cancer (upper endoscopy every 2–3 years), and urinary tract cancers (annual urinalysis).

BIBLIOGRAPHY

1. Syngal S, Brand RE, Church JM, et al. ACG clinical guideline: genetic testing and management of hereditary gastrointestinal cancer syndromes. *Am J Gastroenterol.* 2015;110(2):223-262.
2. Rubenstein JH, Enns R, Heidelbaugh J, Barkun A, Clinical Guidelines Committee. American Gastroenterological Association Institute guideline on the diagnosis and management of Lynch syndrome. *Gastroenterology.* 2015;149(3):777-782.
3. Giardiello FM, Allen JI, Axilbund JE, et al. Guidelines on genetic evaluation and management of Lynch syndrome: a consensus statement by the US Multi-Society Task Force on colorectal cancer. *Gastroenterology.* 2014;147(2):502-526.
4. Hajirawala L, Barton JS. Diagnosis and management of Lynch syndrome. *Dis Colon Rectum.* 2019;62(4):403-405.
5. Sinicrope FA. Lynch syndrome-associated colorectal cancer. *N Engl J Med.* 2018;379(8):764-773.
6. Bresalier RS Colorectal cancer. Sleisenger and Fordtran's Gastrointestinal and Liver Disease. 11th ed. Elsevier; 2020.
7. Qayed E. Gastroenterology Clinical Focus: High yield GI and Hepatology Review- for Boards and Practice. 3rd ed. Independently published; 2022.

ALGORITHM 78.1 Flowchart for the workup and diagnosis of Lynch syndrome after colorectal cancer diagnosis. *IHC,* Immunohistochemistry; *PCR,* polymerase chain reaction.

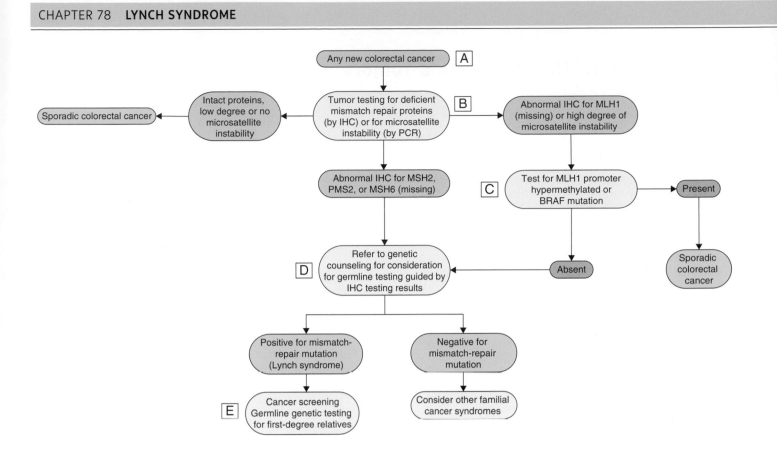

79 Rectal Neuroendocrine Tumors

Emad Qayed

Rectal neuroendocrine tumors are increasing in incidence, and this is likely related to increased use of colonoscopy for colon cancer screening and other indications. The carcinoid syndrome is very uncommon (less than 1%) in patients with rectal neuroendocrine tumors. The risk of metastases from rectal neuroendocrine tumors is related to their size, and ranges from 2%–5% in those smaller than 1 cm (the majority) to about 70% in those that are larger than 2 cm. If a rectal neuroendocrine tumor is suspected during a colonoscopy based on its appearance and rubbery consistency, then it should be marked with endoscopic tattooing, carefully photographed, and endoscopic resection should be attempted. Endoscopic resection can be performed using a variety of methods, including hot snare resection, submucosal injection followed by hot snare resection (endoscopic mucosal resection), and band ligation followed by hot snare resection. Endoscopic full-thickness resection is an emerging technique for the resection of rectal neuroendocrine tumors. The subsequent management approach depends on the size and grade of the tumor and completeness of resection.

A. If the resected tumor is less than 1 cm in size, and complete endoscopic resection was performed and documented during the index colonoscopy, then no further follow-up is required.

B. If endoscopic resection was not confirmed and/or margins are positive on histology, and the lesion is low grade (G1), then flexible sigmoidoscopy should be performed to examine the site of resection. If residual tumor is found, this should be resected endoscopically, and the area marked with endoscopic tattooing (if not previously performed).

C. If tumor size is ≥1 cm, or complete endoscopic resection is not achieved, or the tumor is higher grade (e.g., G2 tumor), the patient should undergo further testing with rectal endoscopic ultrasound (EUS) or magnetic resonance imaging (MRI). The T1 to T4 American Joint Committee on Cancer (AJCC) staging of rectal neuroendocrine tumors is as follows:
T1: Tumor invades the lamina propria or submucosa and is ≤2 cm.
T2: Tumor invades the muscularis propria or is >2 cm with invasion of the lamina propria or submucosa.

T3: Tumor invades through the muscularis propria into subserosal tissue without penetration of overlying serosa.
T4: Tumor invades the visceral peritoneum or other organs or adjacent structures.

D. If the tumor is T1 (≤2 cm), then endoscopic or minimally invasive transanal resection should be performed. No additional follow-up is needed if the tumor is <1 cm in size, while repeat rectal EUS or MRI is recommended if the lesion tumor is between 1 and 2 cm in size.

E. If the tumor is T2–T4, then complete workup with colonoscopy, chest and abdominal imaging, and somatostatin receptor scintigraphy is recommended. Patients with metastatic disease should be managed by surgical or medical therapy based on the size and extent of their primary and metastatic disease.

F. Patients without metastatic disease should undergo surgical resection of the primary tumor followed by periodic clinical follow-up and surveillance by abdominal and pelvic computed tomography (CT) scans.

BIBLIOGRAPHY

1. National Comprehensive Cancer Network (NCCN) Guidelines. Neuroendocrine and Adrenal tumors. Version 1.2022. NCCN.ORG; 2022 [accessed 23.05.22].
2. Meier B, Albrecht H, Wiedbrauck T, Schmidt A, Caca K. Full-thickness resection of neuroendocrine tumors in the rectum. *Endoscopy*. 2020;52(1):68-72. https://doi.org/10.1055/a-1008-9077.
3. Strosberg JR, Al-Toubah T Neuroendocrine tumors. Sleisenger and Fordtran's Gastrointestinal and Liver Disease, 11th Edition, Elsevier, 2021.

ALGORITHM 79.1 Flowchart for the workup and management of rectal neuroendocrine tumors. *CT,* Computed tomography; *EUS,* endoscopic ultrasound; *MRI,* magnetic resonance imaging.

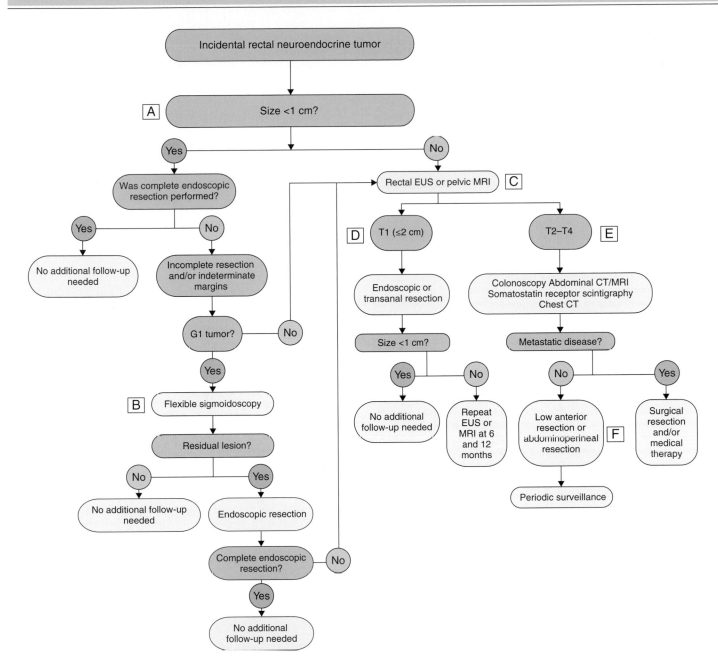

80 Appendiceal Neuroendocrine Tumors

Emad Qayed

Appendiceal neuroendocrine neoplasms are appendiceal epithelial neoplasms with neuroendocrine differentiation and encompass neuroendocrine tumors and neuroendocrine carcinoma. A subset of appendiceal neoplasms are mixed neuroendocrine-nonneuroendocrine neoplasms (MiNENs), which have a neoplastic epithelium with mixed neuroendocrine and nonneuroendocrine components, with each component constituting at least 30% of the neoplasm. Appendiceal neuroendocrine tumors are mostly found incidentally after appendectomy. They are slightly more prevalent in female than in male patients, with an average age of diagnosis of 40–50 years. They account for 0.5%–1% of intestinal neoplasms; and are found in 0.3%–0.9% of appendectomy specimens. Most tumors arise from the tip of the appendix (60%–75%), and less commonly in the body (20%) and base (10%) of the appendix. The majority of tumors are small (<1 cm in diameter) and well differentiated (grade 1). Tumors that are >2 cm in size and are located at the base of the appendix are more likely to present with appendicitis, and are associated with higher rates of lymph node and distant metastases. Of note, the terms "*goblet cell carcinoid*," "*adenocarcinoid*," or "*mixed adenoneuroendocrine carcinoma*" have been previously used to describe a specific type of tumor with neuroendocrine features and adenocarcinoma. These terms are no longer recommended because the World Health Organization has reclassified these tumors as *goblet cell adenocarcinoma*. These tumors are no longer considered a subtype of appendiceal neuroendocrine neoplasms, but rather a subtype of appendiceal adenocarcinoma.

A. If the appendiceal neuroendocrine tumor is diagnosed incidentally upon examination of the appendectomy surgical specimen, further management is dependent on the size of the tumor, its location, and presence of more aggressive histologic features.

B. The majority of tumors ≤1 cm in size are found in the tip or body of the appendix, and have low histologic grade (G1), without mesoappendiceal infiltration. Simple appendectomy is sufficient. For the tumors with more aggressive histologic features (poorly differentiated histology and/or with mesoappendiceal infiltration), or tumors that are located at the base of the appendix, a right hemicolectomy should be considered.

C. For tumors that are 1 to <2 cm in size, cross-sectional imaging with computed tomography (CT) or magnetic resonance imaging (MRI), with or without somatostatin receptor imaging (positron emission tomography [PET] scan or scintigraphy), is recommended to examine for local and distant spread. Simple appendectomy is sufficient in patients without high-risk features.

D. For tumors >2 cm in size, cross-sectional imaging with CT or MRI and somatostatin receptor imaging is recommended. Patients without distant metastasis are managed with right hemicolectomy. Patients with metastatic disease are managed on a case-by-case basis. Treatment includes cytoreductive surgery, liver-directed embolization therapies, and systemic therapy with somatostatin analogs.

BIBLIOGRAPHY

1. Digestive System Tumours. In: WHO Classification of Tumours. 5th ed. Vol 1. IARC, Lyon, 2019.
2. Sleisenger and Fordtran's Gastrointestinal and Liver Disease. 11th ed. Elsevier, 2021 [Chapter 34: Neuroendocrine tumors].
3. Pape UF, Niederle B, Costa F, et al. ENETS consensus guidelines for neuroendocrine neoplasms of the appendix (excluding goblet cell carcinomas). *Neuroendocrinology*. 2016;103(2):144–152.
4. Mohamed A, Wu S, Hamid M, et al. Management of appendix neuroendocrine neoplasms: insights on the current guidelines. *Cancers (Basel)*. 2022;15(1):295. https://doi.org/10.3390/cancers15010295.

ALGORITHM 80.1 Flowchart for the management of neuroendocrine tumors of the appendix. *CT*, Computed tomography; *MRI*, magnetic resonance imaging; *PET*, positron emission tomography.

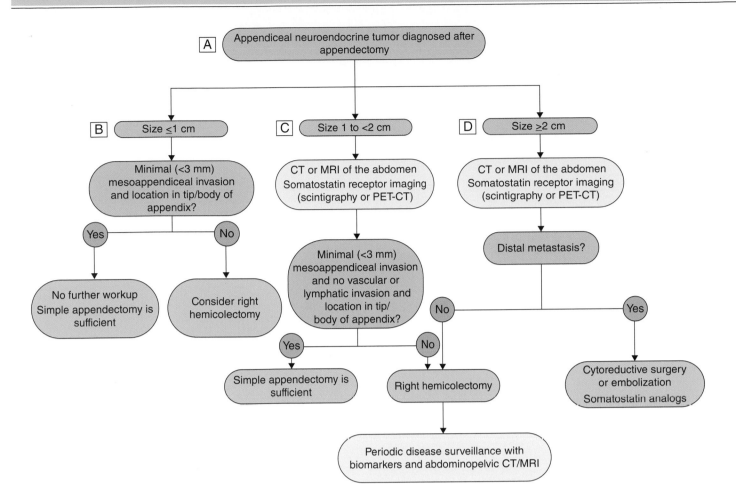

Index